Distinctive Features

Distinctive Features
Theory and Validation

by **Sadanand Singh, Ph.D.**
Professor of Speech and Hearing Sciences
University of Texas Health Science Center at Houston

UNIVERSITY PARK PRESS
BALTIMORE • LONDON • TOKYO

UNIVERSITY PARK PRESS
International Publishers in Science and Medicine
Chamber of Commerce Building
Baltimore, Maryland 21202

Typeset by the Composing Room of Michigan, Inc.
Manufactured in the United States of America by Universal Lithographers, Inc., and The Maple Press Co.

Library of Congress Cataloging in Publication Data

Singh, Sadanand.
Distinctive features.

Includes index.
1. Speech, Disorders of. 2. Distinctive features (Linguistics). 3. Speech perception. 4. Auditory perception. I. Title.
RC423.S53 616.8′55 76-6482
ISBN 0-8391-0754-4

Contents

Preface vii

Concept of Distinctive Features

chapter 1 Basic Concepts 3

chapter 2 Distinctive Feature Systems of Consonants 33
chapter 3 Distinctive Feature Systems of Vowels 75
chapter 4 Comparison of Consonant Feature Systems 89

Role of Distinctive Features in Speech Perception

chapter 5 Distinctive Features in Consonant Perception 101
chapter 6 Distinctive Features in Vowel Perception 147

Role of Distinctive Features in Articulation and Speech Discrimination

chapter 7 Distinctive Features and Language Acquisition (*with a supplemental study by Frederick F. Weiner and John Bernthal*) 155
chapter 8 Distinctive Features in Articulation Deviation 205
chapter 9 Distinctive Features in Auditory Discrimination 233

Index 263

Preface

This book is designed primarily for students and professionals in the fields of speech pathology and audiology. Its goal is to present and promote an understanding of the concept of distinctive features as they relate to speech sounds. The relevancy of distinctive features has been demonstrated in phonological, acoustic, and perceptual analyses of various types of speech in numerous experimental conditions. Distinctive features are presented here as measurable parameters underlying both production and perception of speech. Distinctive features are also discussed for their use in diagnosis and management of speech and hearing problems.

This book is divided into three major sections. The first provides a definition of distinctive features as well as a mapping of how they are used in designating relationships among sounds. Four chapters make up the first section. The first chapter serves as a building block for concepts presented in those that follow. Chapters 2 and 3 present existing distinctive feature systems and discuss their basis. In the fourth chapter, a comparison of the different distinctive feature systems is made with regard to their mutual overlap as well as their dissimilarities. The second section, Chapters 5 and 6, presents historical reviews of relevant perceptual research conducted in the past twenty years. These chapters focus on investigations that test and substantiate the role of distinctive features in the perception of speech sounds.

The final section consists of three chapters that further elaborate upon the role of distinctive features in articulation and speech discrimination, specifically, language acquisition, articulation disorders, and auditory discrimination. In these chapters, studies showing that acquisition of phonemes by children, errors in articulation of phonemes, and phoneme perception by normal and hearing-impaired individuals are based on the parameters of distinctive features.

Although this book is entitled *Distinctive Features: Theory and Validation,* no effort is made in the text to describe a phonological theory from a fixed orientation or allegiance to a given school of linguistic thought. Actually, the section dealing with theory is primarily a systematic development of the distinctive feature hypothesis supported by data substantiating the feature theory.

Readers of this book should gain a keener insight into the relevance of the distinctive feature hypothesis as well as a familiarization with experimental data supporting the feature theory. Students and professionals, especially those in the fields of speech pathology and audiology, should find the literature discussed in this text a source for describing and utilizing distinctive features in the diagnosis and management of speech and hearing problems.

During my work on the manuscript my wife Kala gave many helpful editorial comments and personal encouragement. Acknowledgment is also due Professor Harris Winitz, Pam Curtis, and Fern Waldman, who have read this manuscript and made valuable suggestions.

to Chacha

CONCEPT OF DISTINCTIVE FEATURES

chapter 1
Basic Concepts

CONTENTS

Concept of feature
Concept of phonemic system
Definition of distinctive features
Determining feature specifications of phonemes
Distinctive feature matrix and determination of phoneme differences
Classification of phoneme distinctions
Similarity/dissimilarity hierarchy
Distinctive feature count versus phoneme count
Inequality between feature distinctions
Inter- and intrafeature inequalities
Application to therapy: sample strategies, similarity counts, and competence/performance
Summary

The phoneme is the basic sound unit of a language, and each language has a finite number of them. For example, English has about 45 different phonemes. Although the phoneme is a symbolic entity, its external manifestations may be real, in the sense that they are realized in speaking and listening. The phonetic realization in speaking involves the human speech production mechanisms; e.g., the phoneme /p/ is produced by the approximation of the lips, without vibration of the vocal folds and with the explosion of air. The phonetic realization in listening involves the auditory perception of the speech sounds (phonemes); e.g., the phoneme /p/ normally will be perceived as /p/.

The phoneme is produced by a set of articulatory and phonetic maneuvers that have distinct articulatory and acoustic properties. Both articulatory and acoustic properties are inputs for the perception of the phoneme as a unitary and distinct sound. In order to clarify some basic concepts regarding distinctive features, we will work only with the articulatory property of the phoneme. This aspect is considered crucial in speech production and perception. Also, the features of articulation (labiality, voicing, etc.) are more clearly definable than the acoustic and perceptual features.

CONCEPT OF FEATURE

As humans we have the ability to detect and categorize features. Without these skills we could not observe consistencies among events that might otherwise appear unrelated. The early cognitive growth of young children heavily depends on decisions that involve features. Those features that become important are regarded as distinctive, and those that do not enter into significant perceptual decisions simply go unmentioned.

At some time in a child's perceptual development, he can distinguish between *vertical* and *horizontal* placement. He can later apply this distinction to objects that he has never seen.

For convenience, let us call a vertical object +*vertical* and a horizontal object −*vertical*. Below are vertical and horizontal objects marked appropriately:

+vertical	−vertical	+vertical	−vertical
(*a*)	(*b*)	(*c*)	(*d*)

Objects *a* and *c* are distinctively different from objects *b* and *d*. However, no distinction can be made between objects *a* and *c* and *b* and *d*. To do this we need to add another marker. Let us call this new marker *large*, marked as follows:

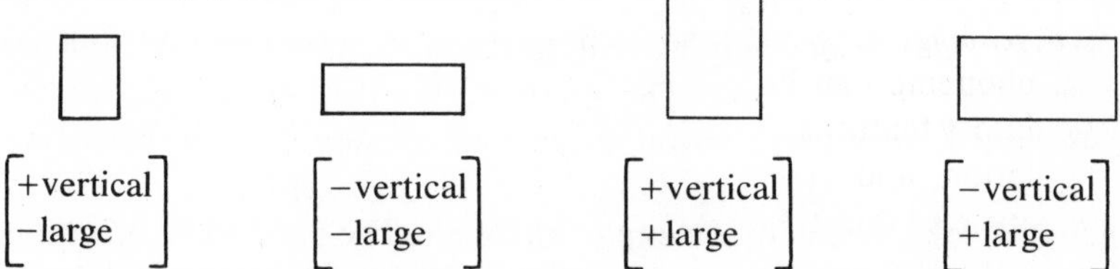

As adults we are able to use the distinctive features of [+vertical] and [+large] with little cognitive strain. Occasionally we encounter difficulty, especially when features are not available for borderline circumstances. For example, at times we may have difficulty in assigning the features[+fat] or [−fat] to our friends and associates. Similarly, linguists do not always agree in their assignment of distinctive features.

CONCEPT OF PHONEMIC SYSTEM

Let us start with the evident and almost axiomatic understanding that the 45 phonemes of the English language are different from one another. The difference between any two phonemes can be established by: 1) determining the parameters possessed by the two phonemes, 2) eliminating the common parameters between the two phonemes, and 3) identifying the parameters not common between them. The similarity between phonemes in terms of the parameters can be best understood by considering two phonemes that have all parameters in common. In this case, the parameter difference between them is zero, and hence they are no longer two different phonemes. On the other hand, two phonemes may be different by a maximum of n parameters, if n parameters are used to describe them. However, in reality it seems that no two phonemes in a language could be different by all n parameters. A phonemic system entails the differing degrees of relationship between the phonemes of a language. As we will see later, in the English phonemic system, which is highly economical, less than one-third of the 45 parameters are used in the description of the English phonemes.

DEFINITION OF DISTINCTIVE FEATURES

An examination of the phonemes of English reveals that, because different phonemes share some attributes and differ by other attributes, only a limited number of attributes are utilized to discriminate a large number of phonemes. Such attributes are called the distinctive features. ***Distinctive features are the physical (articulatory or acoustic) and psychological (perceptual) realities of the phoneme.*** In other words, each phoneme can be described and differentiated in terms of: 1) articulatory features, namely, the place of articulation, the manner of articulation, and voicing; 2) acoustic features, namely, frequency, intensity, and duration of speech sounds; and 3) perceptual features, which are the result of the auditory discrimination between the phonemes. The following discussion deals only with the articulatory features.

DETERMINING FEATURE SPECIFICATIONS OF PHONEMES

Articulatory descriptions such as place of articulation, manner of articulation, and voicing are used to determine the articulatory features of the phonemes of a language. Starting with the place of articulation feature and examining only the English stop phonemes, it is known in classical phonetic theory that the phoneme /p/ is a bilabial stop. The description of bilabiality is also shared by the oral stop /b/ and the nasal stop /m/. Also it is known that the phoneme /t/ is an alveolar stop. This description of alveolarity is also shared by the oral stop /d/ and the nasal stop /n/. Finally, it is known that the phoneme /k/ is a velar stop, and, again, the velarity is shared by the oral stop /g/ and the nasal stop /ŋ/. Thus a set of nine selected English consonants /p, b, m, t, d, n, k, g, ŋ/ shares three places of articulation: bilabial, alveolar, and velar. This set can be further described in terms of the feature manner of articulation. The three consonants /m, n, ŋ/ are nasal, and the remaining six consonants /p, b, t, d, k, g/ are oral. In addition, the set can be described in terms of the feature voicing. The three consonants /p, t, k/ are voiceless and the remaining six /b, d, g, m, n, ŋ/ are voiced.

Thus all nine consonants of the set may be distinguished by a three-feature system, the two binary features (manner and voicing) and a ternary feature (place of articulation). A binary feature has only two specifications, one opposite in nature to the other. For example, the feature voicing may be either +voice or −voice, indicating the presence or absence of vocal fold vibration. In some instances the presence of voicing is denoted by 1 and the absence of voicing by 0. In the specification of manner of articulation, one would mark /m, n, ŋ/ as +nasal or 1 and the remaining consonants of the set as −nasal or 0. The place of articulation is a ternary feature and, therefore, cannot use the binary specifications (+) and (−). Therefore, 0, 1, and 2 specifications can be used, where 0 specifies labiality, 1 specifies alveolarity, and 2 specifies velarity. However, whereas zero voicing (complete lack of vocal fold vibration) and zero nasality (a complete lack of nasal resonance) are conceivable, a zero place of articulation seems inconceivable. Therefore, /p, b, m/ have been described as place-1, /t, d, n/ as place-2, and /k, g, ŋ/ as place-3.

DISTINCTIVE FEATURE MATRIX AND DETERMINATION OF PHONEME DIFFERENCES

As a result of the above description the nine English phonemes under consideration can be now described utilizing three articulatory parameters, as shown in Table 1-1. Consider the second column of this table; the phonemes /p, b, m/ share bilabiality, the phonemes /p, b/ share the oral stop characteristic, and the phonemes /b, m/ share the presence of voicing. In the center column, the phonemes /t, d, n/ share alveolarity, /t, d/ share the oral stop characteristic, and /d, n/ share the presence of voicing. In the next column, the phonemes /k, g, ŋ/ share velarity, /k, g/ share the oral stop characteristic, and /g, ŋ/ share the

Table 1-1. Distinctive feature breakdown of nine English consonants

	Place of articulation			
Manner of articulation	Bilabial	Alveolar	Velar	Voicing
Oral stop	p	t	k	Voiceless
Oral stop	b	d	g	Voiced
Nasal stop	m	n	ŋ	Voiced

presence of voicing. Consider the rows now; the phonemes in the first row share the absence of voicing, the phonemes in the second and third rows share the presence of voicing, and the phonemes in the third row share the presence of nasality.

It is conventional to describe the phonemes in columns and the distinctive features in rows. Thus, the above phonemic system can be described as shown in Table 1-2.

There is a definite advantage to converting the preceding system (Table 1-1) into a matrix of binary and ternary features (Table 1-2). However, although the advantage is practical, some assumptions underlying these conversions may not hold. For example, the assumption that all voiced consonants uniformly have one degree of voicing whereas all voiceless consonants uniformly have the opposite degree of voicing (namely, lack of voicing) may not hold when tested experimentally. Also, the notion that labial, alveolar, and velar stops differ linearly by one step may not be a realistic assumption.

The advantage of a matrix such as that in Table 1-2 is its ability to determine numerically the degree of difference and/or similarity between a pair of phonemes. This eventually would lead to a network of descriptions for a given phoneme set. For the nine phonemes, for example, the maximal number of contrasts would be $n \times (n - 1)/2$ or $9 \times 8/2$ or 36 individual pairs of phonemes. The differences and

Table 1-2. Distinctive feature system involving nine English consonants

	Phoneme specification								
Feature	p	b	t	d	k	g	m	n	ŋ
Voicing	0	1	0	1	0	1	1	1	1
Nasality	0	0	0	0	0	0	1	1	1
Place	1	1	2	2	3	3	1	2	3

similarities among the 36 pairs of phonemes can be determined by counting the distinctive feature differences. The fewer the number of feature differences between a pair of phonemes, the closer the relationship between the phonemes. The greater the number of differences between the phonemes, the farther the relationship.

A sample use of the matrix to determine phonemic interrelationships is the consonant /p/, at the top of the first column in Table 1-2; /p/ may be compared with the consonants at the top of the remaining columns. The basis for comparison is the feature in each of the three rows. It may be noted here that the order in which the nine consonants are arranged is entirely arbitrary, and that no matter in what order they are arranged, the relationship of each consonant to the remaining eight remains unaltered.

The phoneme /p/ is specified as having 0 voice, 0 nasality, and 1 place while the phoneme /b/, with which /p/ is compared, is specified as having 1 voice, 0 nasality, and 1 place. Utilizing these specifications, the relationship between the phonemes /p/ and /b/ can be expressed as follows:

	Voice	*Nasality*	*Place*
/p/ =	(0)	(0)	(1)
/b/ =	(1)	(0)	(1)

where /p/ and /b/ have similar specifications for nasality and place and different specifications for voicing. Thus, /p-b/ is described as being a minimally distinct pair of phonemes. ***A distinction of one feature between a pair of phonemes constitutes a minimally distinct pair.*** Or, stated in another way, /p/ and /b/ constitute a maximally similar pair of phonemes. ***In a set of features (n = 3 in this case), if two sounds are similar by n − 1 features, they are considered maximally similar.*** In the example given above, /p/ and /b/ phonemes are maximally similar because they have $(n - 1)$ or 2 similar feature specifications (both are non-nasal, bilabial consonants).

In comparing /p/ with the rest of the phonemes at the top of the remaining columns, other distinctions based on the same matrix become apparent. The features voicing, nasality, and place are denoted by V, N, and P, respectively, and the specifications 0, 1, 2, and 3 are denoted as superscripts:

$$\text{p/t} = V^0N^0P^1/V^0N^0P^2 = P^1 = 1$$

The result is a *one*-feature difference because of the one-place difference.

$$p/d = V^0N^0P^1/V^1N^0P^2 = VP^1 = 2$$

The result is a *two*-feature difference; the features are voicing and place of articulation.

$$p/k = V^0N^0P^1/V^0N^0P^3 = P^2 = 2$$

The result is two degrees of difference as a result of a difference of two on the place continuum.

$$p/g = V^0N^0P^1/V^1N^0\,P^3 = VP^2 = 3$$

The result is three degrees of difference involving one voicing difference and two place differences.

$$p/m = V^0N^0P^1/V^1N^1P^1 = VN = 2$$

The result is two differences involving the features voicing and nasality.

$$p/n = V^0N^0P^1/V^1N^1P^2 = VNP^1 = 3$$

The result is three differences involving the features voicing, nasality, and place.

$$p/\eta = V^0N^0P^1/V^1N^1P^3 = VNP^2 = 4$$

The result is four degrees of differences involving the features voicing, nasality, and two place differences.

In this manner the interphonemic relationships of the phonemes /b, t, d, k, g, m, n, ŋ/ can also be established.

CLASSIFICATION OF PHONEME DISTINCTIONS

Pairs having a difference of one feature, e.g., /p, b/ and /p, t/, are called minimally distinct pairs; pairs differing by two features, e.g., /p, d/, /p, k/, and /p, m/, are called duply distinct pairs; pairs differing by three features, e.g., /p, g/ and /p, n/, are called triply distinct pairs; and pairs differing by four features, e,g., /p, ŋ/, are called quadruply distinct pairs.

These degrees of differences are very relevant in the realization of phonemes in all modes of encoding and decoding of speech. The sounds of speech are known to be processed in terms of distinctive features. The processing includes speaking, listening, and other modes of speech coding. An examination of the four words /pɪn/, /bɪn/, /tɪn/, and /kɪn/ shows that, although these words differ by one phoneme, they are not all minimally distinct pairs in terms of the three features described above. Therefore, they are referred to as phonemically minimal pairs. ***A phonemically minimal pair is a set of two words that are different by only one phoneme.***

Phonemic and distinctive feature disparities for the same four words are displayed in Table 1-3. Phonemic disparities are counted in terms of the number of phonemes that are different in two words, while distinctive feature disparities are counted in terms of the number of distinctive feature differences between two phonemes. Regarding phonemic disparity, all four words /pɪn/, /bɪn/, /tɪn/, and /kɪn/ differ by one phoneme, all in the initial position. Phonemic comparisons indicate that /pɪn/ is minimally different from /bɪn/, /tɪn/, and /kɪn/ as /p/ is minimally different from /b/, /t/, and /k/. The same is true for the remaining comparison.

Although phonemic disparity is 1 in all cases, distinctive feature disparity ranges from 1 to 3, as can be observed from this table. Distinctive feature comparisons indicate that /p/ differs from /b/ and /t/ by one feature and from /k/ by two features; /b/ differs from /t/ by two features and from /k/ by three features; and /t/ differs from /k/ by one feature. The distinctive feature relationship between these four arbitrarily chosen English stop phonemes enables one to predict that, because /bɪn/ is minimally distinct from /pɪn/, it would be most frequently erred with /pɪn/ in production and perception. Since /bɪn/ is duply distinct from /tɪn/, the second most frequent error in production or perception would be with /tɪn/, and since /bɪn/ is triply distinct from /kɪn/, the least frequent production substitution or perceptual confusion would occur between /bɪn/ and /kɪn/. Thus, on the basis that /bɪn/

Table 1-3. Comparison of phonemic and distinctive feature disparities

Phonemic disparity			Word	Distinctive feature disparity		
			pin			
		1	bin	1		
	1	1	tin	1	2	
1	1	1	kin	2	3	1

is different from /pɪn/ by one feature and from /tɪn/ and /kɪn/ by two and three features, respectively, it can be concluded that /bɪn/ is more similar to /pɪn/ than it is to /tɪn/ and /kɪn/, and also that /bɪn/ is more similar to /tɪn/ than it is to /kɪn/.

It is important to note here that distinctive features generally are classificatory in nature because they are classes of attributes that apply to a group of phonemes. Some phonemes share many of these features, others share few, and still others share none. ***When a group of speech sounds can be designated by fewer features than any individual member of that group, the group is referred to as a natural class. If a group of phonemes shows no commonality of features, it is referred to as an unnatural class.*** In articulatory and perceptual decisions of speakers and listeners, it is safe to assume that most errors occur between the phonemes of a natural class and errors seldom occur between the phonemes of an unnatural class. For example, there will be greater errors between the sounds within the oral stop category and no errors between the sounds in the oral stop and vowel categories.

The preceding discussion of the interphonemic relationships is extremely useful in the understanding of phonemes. On the basis of these relations it can be concluded that: 1) phonemes are interrelated in terms of distinctive features, 2) the interrelationships of the phonemes are of differing degree, and 3) these relationships reflect on phoneme production, phoneme perception, and other processes involved in the encoding and decoding of speech.

SIMILARITY/DISSIMILARITY HIERARCHY

Given the nine phonemes in the set of stop consonants, a hierarchy of relationships can be developed utilizing the three distinctive articulatory features that were used to discern them. In the paradigm below, the phoneme preceding the arrow is the one being compared, and the phonemes following the arrow are the remainder phonemes of the set ($n - 1$, or eight in this instance) arranged in order of their relative degrees of relationship. The nearer the phoneme is to the one that it is being compared with, the closer the relationship is. In the event that more than one phoneme has an identical number of differences from the phoneme being compared, then they are parallelly listed. For example, if the phoneme to be compared is /p/, then of the nine consonants two, namely /b/ and /t/, would be shown closest to it. The next sets of phonemes to follow would be /d/, /k/, and /m/, followed by /g/ and /n/, finally followed by /ŋ/. Thus the relationship of /p/ to the remaining eight phonemes of the set can be presented as:

$$\text{/p/} \rightarrow \left\{\begin{matrix}\text{/b/}\\ \text{/t/}\end{matrix}\right\} \left\{\begin{matrix}\text{/d/}\\ \text{/k/}\\ \text{/m/}\end{matrix}\right\} \left\{\begin{matrix}\text{/g/}\\ \text{/n/}\end{matrix}\right\} \left\{\text{/ŋ/}\right\}$$

where the first set of consonants following the arrow is minimally distinct, the second set duply distinct, the third set triply distinct, and the fourth set quadruply distinct.

Use of Tree Diagram

A tree diagram, such as that shown in Figure 1-1, demonstrates the relevance of the above relationships in generative terms. The diagram utilizes step-function rules where each step is made of a minimally distinct pair. In Figure 1-1, starting with the phoneme /p/, /b/ is minimally distinct for voicing and /t/ is minimally distinct for place. The phoneme /b/ generates /m/ and /d/ because both /m/ and /d/ are minimally distinct from /b/. The phoneme /t/ generates /d/ and /k/ because they are minimally distinct from /t/. Further, /m/ generates /n/, and /d/ generates /n/, because both /m/ and /d/ are minimally distinct from /n/. /d/ also generates /g/, just as /k/ generates /g/, because both /d/ and /k/ are minimally distinct from /g/. Finally, /n/ and /g/ generate /ŋ/ because they are each minimally distinct from /ŋ/.

This tree diagram reflects four levels of feature differences from the phoneme /p/ and the generative structure of the other eight phonemes of the set. Following any one branch, a minimal distinct hierarchy can be established for the nine phonemes. Examining the branches from left to right, the branch at the extreme left hand indicates that /p/ is minimally distinct from /b/ (for voicing), /b/ from /m/ (for nasality), /m/ from /n/ (for place), and /n/ from/ŋ/ (for place). The next branching shows that /p/ is minimally distinct from /b/ (for voicing), /b/ from /d/ (for place), /d/ from /n/ (for nasality), and again

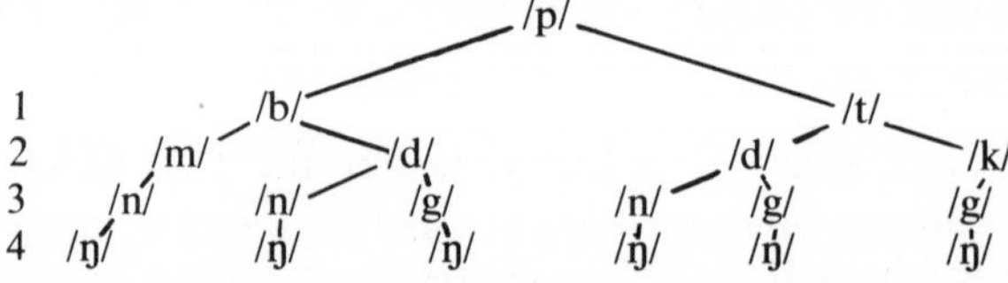

Figure 1-1. A tree diagram illustrating the hierarchical interrelationships between nine phonemes.

/n/ from /ŋ/ (for place). The next branch shows that /p/ is different from /b/, /d/, /g/, and /ŋ/ in the hierarchy, where /p/ is different from /b/ (for voicing), /b/ from /d/ (for place), /d/ from /g/ (for place), and /g/ from /ŋ/ (for nasality). The next branch to the right shows that /p/ is minimally distinct from /t/ (for place), /t/ from /d/ (for voicing), /d/ from /n/ (for nasality), and /n/ from /ŋ/ (for place). The next branch shows the /p/, /t/, /d/, /g/, /ŋ/ branching, where /p/ is one feature different from /t/ (for place), /t/ from /d/ (for voicing), /d/ from /g/ (for place), and /g/ from /ŋ/ (for nasality). Finally, the branching to the extreme right shows the /p/, /t/, /k/, /g/, /ŋ/ branching where /p/ is minimally distinct from /t/ (for place), /t/ from /k/ (for place), /k/ from /g/ (for voicing), and /g/ from /ŋ/ (for nasality).

The basis of this tree diagram is the consonant-by-feature matrix (Table 1-2) that distinctively specifies the nine consonants of the set in terms of the three distinctive features: voicing, nasality, and place. The purpose of this diagram is to demonstrate the hierarchy of relationships among the four arbitrarily selected phonemes of English /p/, /b/, /t/, and /k/ in the words /pin/, /bin/, /tin/, and /kin/. The most important function of a diagram such as the one presented in Figure 1 is to demonstrate the alternative strategies that a speaker or listener may adopt in the realization of these phonemes. The number and type of features present in the repertoire of a speaker or a listener determine the type and number of alternatives that he may use.

Sample Speaker Problems

The generative hierarchy of the relationships of /p/ to /b/, /t/, and /k/ phonemes indicates that, all things being equal, a speaker would substitute /p/ for /b/ if the feature voicing (+voicing to be precise) were weak or absent in the speaker's repertoire. In the instance of a child learning language, the feature voicing might not yet have been acquired, and the child would typically refer to "big" as "pig." A listener also would make such substitutions when acoustic parameters that distinguish the voiceless/voice contrast in labials have been grossly distorted, either in the auditory stimulus or when the listener is incapable of hearing the distinction.

A second speaker who substitutes /p/ for /t/ has kept intact (preserved or retained) the voicing feature; the error is attributable to the feature place of articulation. Again, in the event that a child is learning the language, the place of articulation distinction may not be present in his productive repertoire. These two speakers, one who has the p/b substitution and another who has the p/t substitution, demonstrate that, because in both instances minimally distinct phonemes have been replaced, each speaker's productive repertoire has a "very minor" problem.

A third speaker of the English language who substitutes /p/ for /m/ cannot be considered as having a minor substitution problem. The reason is that this speaker probably has not acquired in his phonetic repertoire the phonemes /b/ and /n/, which are the nearest of the relations to /m/. A substitution of /p/ for /m/ indicates a two-feature difference, i.e., that of voicing and nasality. As has been described earlier, the feature ingredients of /m/ are +voice, +nasal, and place-1. The closest approximation of these ingredients would involve the substitutions made by sounds having any two of the three ingredients present in the substitutions. Thus, within the minimally different paradigm, there are three possible substitutions:

1. −Voice, +nasal, and place-1 = not possible in English
2. +Voice, −nasal, and place-1 = /b/
3. +Voice, +nasal, and place-2 = /n/

Actually, in the English language there are only two possible substitutions where two parameters (attributes or features) are retained and only one erred. In the substitution of /p/ for /m/ two of the three features were erred. Therefore, this speaker may be considered as having a greater substitution problem than the other two speakers. However, this speaker must be given credit for maintaining the similarity of the feature place of articulation. Although his errors are on the voicing and nasality dimensions, he has identified the place of articulation correctly. However, his production repertoire is better than that of speakers who have a three- or four-feature problem.

Let us consider a fourth speaker who substitutes /p/ for /n/. His errors involve: 1) voicing, because /p/ is a voiceless sound and /n/ is voiced; 2) nasality, because /p/ is non-nasal and /n/ is nasal; and 3) place of articulation, because /p/ is place-1 and /n/ is place-2. Thus, in a three-feature system consisting of voicing, nasality, and place of articulation, this speaker is substituting voiceless for voiced, non-nasal for nasal, and place-1 for place-2. Therefore, for all evaluative purposes, this speaker may be considered as having a "very serious" problem with the sound system of English. There is one aspect of this substitution for which the speaker may be given credit. The error involves the substitution of place-1 for place-2 rather than the substitution of place-1 for place-3. It is generally considered that, other things being equal, place-1 is more similar to place-2 than to place-3.

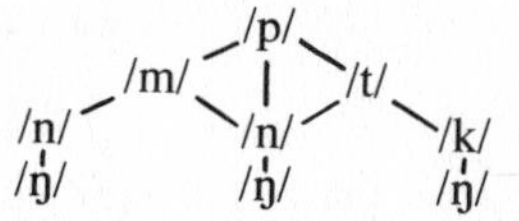

/p/
/m/ /t/
/n/ /n/ /k/
/ŋ/ /ŋ/ /ŋ/

Figure 1-2. A tree diagram illustrating the productive repertoire of a speaker who substitutes /p/ for /b/.

Thus, it may be concluded that, although the speaker substituting /p/ for /n/ has much greater problems than the one who substitutes /p/ for /m/, his problem is not as great as that of the speaker who might substitute /p/ for /ŋ/—a case of maximal dissimilarity (voicing, nasality, and two place differences) and an "extremely serious" problem.

The tree diagram presented for a normal speaker of the English language (Figure 1-1) also can be presented for each of the five speakers chosen for illustrating the notion of dissimilarity/similarity hierarchy. However, it is not safe to draw a diagram on the basis of one substitution alone. For example, speakers who substitute /p/ for /m/, /p/ for /n/, and /p/ for /ŋ/ apparently would have many more substitutions in their repertoire. Tree diagrams for the two speakers who made minimally distinct substitutions are drawn in Figures 1-2 and 1-3 to show that the voicing problem in the former and the place of articulation problem in the latter cut across the total productive repertoire of these speakers.

It may be pointed out that it is assumed in Figures 1-2 and 1-3 that a speaker's substitution is in terms of features and not phonemes. Thus, if a speaker substitutes /p/ for /t/, he is understood to have a problem with the feature place of articulation (place-2), and it is deduced that he may have all alveolars (place-2 sounds) absent from his productive repertoire. It is assumed that, because he substitutes /p/ for /t/, he would substitute /b/ for /d/ and /m/ for /n/. Similarly, it is assumed in the instance of the speaker who substitutes /p/ for /b/ that his productive repertoire does not include voiced consonants. Thus, his substitution may entail /p/ for /b/, /t/ for /d/, and /k/ for /g/.

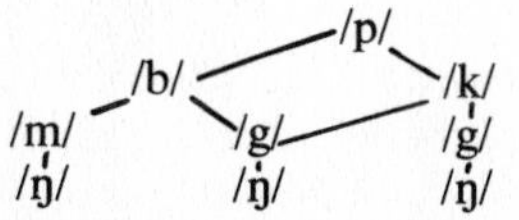

/p/
/b/ /k/
/m/ /g/ /g/
/ŋ/ /ŋ/ /ŋ/

Figure 1-3. A tree diagram illustrating the productive repertoire of a speaker who substitutes /p/ for /t/.

DISTINCTIVE FEATURE COUNT VERSUS PHONEME COUNT

Counting errors in terms of distinctive features is a more representative indicator of the magnitude of a speaker's problem than counting the aggregate of the phonemes. Although counting substitution errors in terms of phonemes entails the tallying of *each* additional error for each substitution, counting distinctive features means considering as *one* all errors pertaining to a feature. In the instance of the speaker who substitutes /p/ for /b/ and, therefore, is considered to have the voicing problem, additional errors or substitutions in his productive repertoire that involve voicing alone are not counted as additional errors. Thus, for example, although the phonemic count would tally three different errors for substitutions of /b, d, g/ by /p, t, k/, respectively, the distinctive feature count would consider them all as one voicing error.

The principles underlying the above assumption are that sounds of a language are interrelated in terms of the parameters that are involved in their production, and that if a parameter of production is not realized according to the established conventions of the language, then that error should be related to the parameter and not to the individual sounds. In other words, errors of articulation of these nine phonemes involve errors of the three distinctive features and do not constitute nine separate problems.

In terms of the acquisition of English phonology or the teaching of the sounds of speech to articulatorily deviant children, it may be emphasized that the distinctive feature system approach marks a considerable departure from the phoneme count approach. In the normal learning of phonology, a child may not acquire all the voiced/voiceless contrasts at the same time; however, if he has acquired one contrast, there is the competence in the phonological repertoire of that child to acquire the remaining contrasts in a relatively short period of time. Similarly, in articulation therapy, if a child has shown a voicing problem then the therapist should concentrate on the feature voicing and not on the teaching of each individual sound.

For example, in the instance of the substitution of /p, t, k/ for /b, d, g/, respectively, it would not make sense to say that the child has a /b/ problem, a /d/ problem, and a /g/ problem. The child really does not have three different problems; there are no individual "/b/" problems, "/d/" problems, or "/g/" problems per se. In saying that a child has a /b/ problem, one implies that he has problems with the parameters or the features of /b/. A close examination of the child's phonemic system would reveal at once that he does not have a /b/ problem but only a fraction (one-third) of the so-called problem. Similarly, his so-called /d/ and /g/ problems are each one-third problems because in both cases only one feature (voicing) has been erred.

A question that may be asked here is: Are the different cases of voicing errors additive? Not necessarily. Actually, −voice has been found to be of different importance than +voice both in speech production and speech perception. A voicing problem may involve the substitution of a −voicing consonant for a +voice consonant (e.g., a substitution of /p/ for /b/) or the substitution of a +voice consonant for a −voice consonant (e.g., a substitution of /b/ for /p/). In the further deliberations of these features, it will be necessary to deal with the substitution of a minus feature specification for a plus feature specification apart from the substitution of a plus specification for a minus specification. At this point, however, they are both described as the feature voicing. Thus, a −nasal substitution for a +nasal (e.g., /d/ for /n/ or /b/ for /m/) as well as a +nasal substitution for a −nasal consonant (e.g., /n/ for /d/ and /m/ for /b/) are all denoted as nasality problems.

If there were only a set of nine consonants in the English language as described in Table 1-2, all substitutions that a speaker would make would involve only the three features and their different combinations. Of the 36 possible contrasts formed by the nine arbitrarily chosen consonants, 12 pairs have one feature difference between them, 14 pairs have two feature differences between them, eight pairs have three feature differences between them, and two pairs have four feature differences between them. As has been indicated earlier, the speaker whose substitutions are limited to a one-feature difference can be considered to have a smaller magnitude of articulatory or discrimination error than the speaker whose substitutions are two features different, and so on. Twelve of the total 36 pairs of consonants that are considered different by one feature (minimally distinct pairs) are: /p, t/, /p, b/, /t, k/, /t, d/, /k, g/, /b, d/, /b, m/, /d, g/, /d, n/, /g, ŋ/, /m, n/, and /n, ŋ/. The 14 pairs of consonants that are different by two features (duply distinct) are: /p, k/, /p, d/, /p, m/, /t, b/, /t, n/, /k, d/, /t, g/, /k, ŋ/, /b, g/, /b, n/, /d, m/, /d, ŋ/, /g, n/, and /m, ŋ/. The eight pairs of consonants that are different by three features (triply distinct) are: /p, g/, /p, n/, /t, m/, /t, ŋ/, /k, b/, /k, n/, /b, ŋ/, and /g, m/. The two pairs of consonants that are four features different (quadruply distinct) are /k, m/ and /p, ŋ/.

INEQUALITY BETWEEN FEATURE DISTINCTIONS

In the above example, of the 12 pairs of minimally distinct consonants, three of the distinctions are attributable to the feature voicing (/p-b, t-d, k-g/), three are attributable to the feature nasality (/b-m, d-n, g-ŋ/), and six are attributable to the feature place of articulation (/p-t, t-k, b-d, d-g, m-n, n-ŋ/). The question that follows is: Do these three features distinguish the phonemes equitably? In other words, can the minimal distinction attributable to voicing be treated equal to the minimal distinction attributable to the place of articulation or the minimal distinction attributable to nasality?

On the surface, it seems logical to assume that, because the distinction of /p, b/, /p, t/, and /b, m/ in each case can be computed to result in a one-feature difference, there is equality between the three features. However, this is not true. The different features of the above example carry differing production strategies and hence have differing degrees of importance in speaking and discriminating English phonemes. For example, in general, the minimal distinction attributable to the feature nasality may be considered more firm (or difficult to obliterate) than the minimal distinction attributable to the feature voicing. The minimal distinction attributable to the feature voicing may be considered more firm than the minimal distinction attributable to the feature place of articulation. This may explain why children's speech production errors have the greatest number of place of articulation errors. The obliteration of the feature nasality would involve the inability on the part of a native English speaker to keep apart the oral cavity from the nasal cavity. The distinction of oral/nasal is not a very fine one, and unless the speaker has a velopharyngeal anomaly he should produce this distinction easily. Incidentally, the oral/nasal distinction is one of the earliest distinctions learned in most languages of the world.

For the obliteration of the feature voicing, a speaker or a listener would have to mistake the presence of vocal fold vibration for the absence of vibration, and vice versa. The speaker or listener who makes such an error may have greater problems than the one who makes an error on the continuum of place of articulation. In English, the minimal distinction attributable to the feature place of articulation, in all instances except labials, involves the placement of the different portions of the tongue on the continuum of the palate. There is a very systematic variation of the body of the tongue as it makes its contact with the teeth, alveolar ridge, hard palate, and velum. Going from front to back and examining only one representative sound for a given place of articulation, the following configurations of the contact of tongue body with the different areas of the lips, teeth, hard palate, and velum are possible in English:

Both lips	/b/	(1)
Lower lip/upper front teeth	/v/	
Tongue tip/front teeth	/ð/	
Tongue tip/alveolar ridge	/d/	(2)
Frontal part of the tongue/hard palate	/dʒ/	
Back of the tongue/soft palate (velum)	/g/	(3)

Among these six representations of the place of articulation feature in the English language, the stop consonants are realized only at three places. Because currently we are dealing with only a set of nine English oral and nasal stops, it may be convenient for us to view the place of articulation as a ternary feature system represented by: 1) both lips, 2) tongue tip and alveolar ridge, and 3) back of the tongue and soft palate (velum).

Motor and Sensory Correlates

The relations of the tongue to the places it contacts (tongue tip to alveolar ridge and back of the tongue to velum) can be altered with ease. The relation of the tongue to the place of articulation is explained in Table 1-4, which shows that, given the separations of the tongue into front and back portions and the separations of the palate also into front and back portions, only the front of the tongue contacts the front of the palate and only the back of the tongue contacts the back of the palate. Although the tongue is an elastic body and can easily approximate the lips, in normal circumstances it does not intervene with the production of bilabial stops. However, during a faulty production strategy, it may not be difficult for the tongue to alter its activities. Within the front-of-the-tongue category as well as within the back-of-the-tongue category, consonants are more vulnerable to production errors.

For motor controls, the alveolar ridge and velum cannot be compared because: 1) there is no motor movement of the alveolar ridge per se, and 2) both the front two-thirds and back one-third of the tongue are driven by the same motor command (hypoglossal nerve). From the point of view of the motor nerve, the anterior and posterior portions of the tongue are driven by the same nerve, namely, the hypoglossal (12th cranial) nerve. That is, the portion of the tongue

Table 1-4. Motor and sensory correlates to lips, alveolar ridge, velum, and anterior and posterior portions of the tongue

	Lips	Alveolar ridge	Anterior two-thirds of the tongue	Velum	Posterior one-third of the tongue
Motor	Facial n.	—	Hypoglossal n.	Pharyngeal plexis of vagus n.; glossopharyngeal n.; accessory n.; trigeminal n. to the tensor veli palatini m.	Hypoglossal n.
Sensory	Trigeminal n.	Trigeminal n.	Facial n.; Glossopharyngeal n. (taste); trigeminal n. (for all other senses)	Glossopharyngeal n.; palatine branch of trigeminal n.	Glossopharyngeal n. (taste and sensory)

responsible for the production of /d/ and the portion responsible for the production of /g/ are innervated by the same nerve. The sensory controls, however, show that, although the alveolar ridge and its tongue correlate (the front of the tongue) are supplied by the trigeminal (5th cranial) nerve, the velum and its tongue correlate (the back of the tongue) are supplied by the glossopharyngeal (9th cranial) nerve.

Thus, in neuromotor terms, the difference between /d/ and /g/ (a minimal distinction attributable to the feature place of articulation) mainly results from the sensory differences between the trigeminal and glossopharyngeal nerves. The distinction of /b/ from /d/ is clear on the motor nerve continuum (/b/, involving the lips driven by the facial (7th cranial) nerve, and /d/, involving the front of the tongue driven by the hypoglossal nerve). However, on the sensory continuum the same (trigeminal) nerve supplies the lips and the alveolar ridge. Thus, /b/ is different from /d/ because of motor and not sensory controls while /d/ is different from /g/ because of sensory and not motor controls.

The focal point of the foregoing discussion is to indicate that, *although two pairs of phonemes may differ by one feature each, the magnitude of those differences may not be considered equal.* Although the minimal distinction attributable to nasality, voicing, and place of articulation may yield one difference each, the difference of nasality is not equal to the difference of voicing, and the difference of voicing is not equal to the difference of place of articulation.

Numerical Weightings

One of the advantages of interrelating phonemes in terms of features is the numerical output of the differences. However, since the different *one*-feature differences are not equal, it is only with great care that one can add these differences linearly. Given that nasality is stronger than voicing, and voicing stronger than place (strength of a feature is denoted by the ability of the feature not to be obliterated or lost easily), a combination of one difference of nasality and one difference of place would be stronger than a combination of one degree of voicing and one degree of place of articulation. For example, although the differences between the phoneme pairs /p-m/ and /p-d/ are of two features each (/p/ is different from /m/ because of nasality and voicing and is different from /d/ because of voicing and place), it would be much more difficult to diminish the distinction of the /p-m/ pair than it would be of the /p-d/ pair.

We can draw similar conclusions regarding the triple and quadruple differences between pairs of phonemes. Just as the *one*-feature difference by a given feature is not equal to the *one*-feature difference by another feature, the two-, three-, and four-feature differences by given combinations of features may not all be equal. The foregoing example of the /p-m/ contrast compared with the /p-d/ contrast exemplifies the above statement.

Application

Although there may be enough evidence presented by now to disappoint the reader regarding the economy, unambiguity, and simplicity of the distinctive feature model, it may be pointed out that these constraints are developed to account more realistically for the problems of phoneme production and perception. The hierarchy developed to ascertain the relative strength of the features would be relevant in determining the normal phonological development and also in ascertaining the magnitude of the articulatory problems in different children. For example, the child who has a p/m substitution may be a more severe case of misarticulation than the child who has a p/d problem, simply because the p/m subsitution indicates errors involving features that are quite resistant but the p/d substitution indicates a loss of features that are not so resistant to obliteration. If the distinctive features are considered as pillars of distinction standing between two phonemes, the pillars of nasality and voicing would be much stronger and, therefore, more difficult to be disregarded. However, if a speaker disregards those pillars in his perception or production, he then apparently has greater problems.

INTER- AND INTRAFEATURE INEQUALITIES

Intrafeature Inequality (Inequality of Feature Specifications)

Actually, before determining the inequality of the minimally distinct pairs of phonemes (interfeature inequality), it is necessary to discuss the inequality of various specifications of a given feature (intrafeature inequality).

A given feature, e.g., voicing, is an aggregate representation of its two opposite specifications: 1) +voice specification, and 2) −voice specification. For the feature place of articulation, the specifications are place-1, place-2, and place-3. Although it is known through some current research that different specifications of a given feature may not have equal weight in the production and perception of speech, in most instances a feature is described as though its different specifications were equitable. In describing the phonological development of a child, it is common to make a statement such as "he has not mastered voicing." When such a statement is made, it is difficult to determine whether the specification the child has not mastered is −voicing or +voicing.

In order to isolate the stage of phonological development in children, it is important not only to describe acquisition in terms of features but also in terms of feature specifications. Different feature specifications employ different aspects of a given speech production mechanism. For example, +voicing involves the vibrations of the vocal cords whereas −voicing involves lack of vibrations; +nasality involves the opening of the nasopharynx whereas −nasality involves the closing of the nasopharynx; and place-1 involves bilabiality, place-2 involves alveolarity, and place-3 involves velarity. It is safe to assume that the different aspects of a given continuum may be mastered at different times and with differing ease in the normal phonological development and, therefore, may require differing habilitative ease in articulation therapy.

It is important to examine the various specifications of a feature when a lack of mastery of that feature exists in a speaker's or listener's system. To say that a feature has been mastered is to imply that both the plus and the minus specifications have been mastered. However, in the instance of the lack of mastery of a feature, three distinctly relevant possibilities exist: 1) the minus specification has not been mastered, 2) the plus specification has not been mastered, and 3) neither the minus nor the plus specification has been mastered. In the instance of a ternary feature, there are seven possibilities: 1) labiality not mastered, 2) alveolarity not mastered, 3) velarity not mastered, 4) labiality and alveolarity not mastered, 5) alveolarity and velarity not mastered, 6) labiality and velarity not mastered, and finally 7) none of the three specifications (labiality, velarity, alveolarity) mastered. Again, in order for a place of articulation feature to be correctly realized in speech production and/or speech perception, none of the seven error possibilities should occur. Both the plus and minus feature specifications cannot be absent simultaneously if there is any speech at all. However, total substitution of feature specification (i.e., a plus specification replaced by a minus specification, and vice versa) is possible.

It is common knowledge that different feature specifications appear in a child's productive repertoire at different times and that a feature is considered acquired only when all its specifications are realized without error. The possibilities of having one specification present while the other is absent can be seen in Table 1-5. In the productive or the perceptual processes, if a speaker or a listener replaces one phoneme by another phoneme, his error in replacement may be of either the plus or the minus specification. In the instance of a binary feature, both the +voice and the −voice error cannot occur simultaneously.

Interfeature Inequality
(Inequality of Minimally Distinct Phoneme Pairs)

The breakdown of 14 minimally distinct pairs of oral stops resulting from the six English oral stops /p, t, k, b, d, g/ is shown in Table 1-5. Fourteen different possibilities exist in the description of the errors that may occur during the course of normal language learning or beyond the stages of normal language learning. In the latter instance, the errors will be labeled as an "articulation problem." In Table 1-5, whether /p/ substitutes /b/ or /b/ substitutes /p/, place-1 has been realized correctly. However, in the substitution of /b/ by /p/ the feature specification +voice is erred whereas in the substitution of /p/ by /b/ the feature specification −voice has been erred. Similarly, in

Table 1-5. Breakdown of feature specifications involving minimally distinct pairs of oral stops

Substitutions of minimal distinction	Acquired feature specification	Unacquired feature specification	Substituted feature
p/b	Place-1	+Voice	−Voice
b/p	Place-1	−Voice	+Voice
t/d	Place-2	+Voice	−Voice
d/t	Place-2	−Voice	+Voice
k/g	Place-3	+Voice	−Voice
g/k	Place-3	−Voice	+Voice
t/k	−Voice	Place-3	Place-2
k/t	−Voice	Place-2	Place-3
b/d	+Voice	Place-2	Place-1
d/b	+Voice	Place-1	Place-2
d/g	+Voice	Place-3	Place-2
g/d	+Voice	Place-2	Place-3
p/t	−Voice	Place-2	Place-1
t/p	−Voice	Place-1	Place-2

both t/d and d/t substitutions, place-2 has been realized correctly. Whereas in the substitution of /d/ by /t/ the +voice is in error, in the substitution of /t/ by /d/ the −voice is in error. In the k/g and g/k substitutions, again, while place-3 has been realized correctly, in the first instance it is a +voice error and in the second instance it is a −voice error. Differing from the above examples, the t/k and the k/t substitutions indicate that, although the feature −voice has been correctly realized, place-3 is in error in the instance of the substitution of /k/ by /t/, while place-2 is erred in the substitution of /t/ by /k/. For the b/d and the d/b substitutions, although the +voice specification is correctly realized, the first instance involves a place-2 error and second instance involves a place-1 error. For the d/g and the g/d substitutions, again, the + specification of the feature voicing is correct. The error is in the incorrect realization of place-3 in the first pair and place-2 in the second pair.

Table 1-5 shows how one or the other value of a feature may be in error and yet the error normally would be labeled in terms of that feature name only. In the p/b substitution it is the +voice that is erred whereas in the b/p substitution it is the −voice that is erred. Yet both errors are described as voicing errors. Research in the areas of phonological acquisition and articulation problems shows that, when there is a voicing error, there is a greater probability that −voice will replace +voice rather than vice versa. Thus, an examination of the substitution patterns of a child with deviant articulation may show greater p/b type substitutions than the b/p type. Similar statements can be made regarding the specifications of the feature place of articulation. Although there is no clear evidence of the relative superiority of the place-2 and place-3 specifications, the evidence is clearly present, both in the language development data and in the patterns of articulatory errors of children, that place-1 is erred less frequently than place-2 or place-3. Recent evidence regarding the hierarchy of the place feature suggests that, within a given manner of articulation (e.g., stops), place-3 is substituted more frequently by place-2 than vice versa, and place-2 is substituted more frequently by place-1 than vice versa. Place-1 is rarely replaced (Singh and Frank, 1972).

Markedness The concepts that one given specification of a feature is learned more easily than another, and that one given specification of a feature replaces the other more frequently than vice versa, have been explained by the term *markedness*. The specifications of a feature can be described in terms of markedness. Given that a feature is binary, one of its specifications may be unmarked and the other marked. Markedness applies only to the articulatory features because its definition implies articulatory parameters. ***A specification is considered unmarked if the articulatory gestures involved in its production are less complex than its marked counterpart.*** Thus, for the feature voicing, −voice is considered unmarked and +voice is considered marked. The reasoning is that, for consonants, +voice necessitates an additional phonetic gesture, namely, the quasivibration of the vocal folds, while −voice lacks this complexity. For the feature nasality, −nasal is unmarked because +nasal has an additional articulatory gesture, the opening of the nasopharyngeal port. For the feature place of articulation, place-1 is unmarked because it involves fewer maneuvers of the articulatory structures as compared to place-2, which is marked. Place-2, in turn, may be considered unmarked when compared to place-3, which is considered marked. As has been mentioned earlier, markedness applies when a comparison is made between any two specifications of a feature. The unmarked specification of a feature is considered easy to produce, easy to learn, and replaces the marked member of a feature more frequently than vice versa. Also, the members of a marked pair, e.g., /b-d/, are considered closer to each other in production and perception than are the members of its parallel unmarked pair /p-t/.

The markedness principle on the one hand accounts for the fact that labial replaces alveolar more frequently than vice versa, voiceless replaces voiced more frequently than vice versa, and non-nasal replaces nasal more frequently than vice versa, and on the other hand accounts for the greater number of replacements within the marked category than within the unmarked. Thus, +nasal replaces +nasal more than −nasal replaces −nasal, and +voice replaces +voice more than −voice replaces −voice.

The marked feature specification is conventionally denoted by *M*, and the unmarked specification is denoted by *U*. The breakdown of the feature specifications in terms of markedness for the arbitrarily chosen nine English stop consonants is shown in Table 1-6. On the place continuum all front consonants (place-1 and place-2) are considered unmarked and the back consonants (place-3) are considered marked. There is evidence in the articulation literature to support this assignment of notation.

With this added intrafeature inequality plus the interfeature inequality discussed earlier, any conclusion regarding the distinctive features must be made in specific terms. The distinctive feature

Table 1-6. Descriptions of feature specifications in terms of markedness

Consonant	Feature specification[a]		
	Voicing	Nasality	Place
p	U	U	U
b	M	U	U
t	U	U	U
d	M	U	U
k	U	U	M
g	M	U	M
m	M	M	U
n	M	M	U
ŋ	M	M	M

[a]M, marked; U, unmarked.

approach would work better than the phonetic approach even if one did not account for the inter- and intrafeature inequalities. However, it would work more precisely if the relative weights or the importance of the specifications of a given feature as well as the differences between the features themselves were taken into account while analyzing, diagnosing, and correcting a given articulatory pattern of a native speaker.

Similarity Hierarchy In spite of the inter- and intrafeature inequalities, it may be safe to say that, in general, a minimally distinct pair of phonemes is closer together in production/perception (therefore easily confused) than a pair of phonemes with two feature differences, and so on. Implicit in this statement is the assumption that no matter how strong a feature is, the difference between two phonemes attributable to that feature is always smaller than the difference between two phonemes attributable to the sum of two features (no matter how weak those two features are):

$$f.x + f.y \geq f.z$$

where $f.x$ and $f.y$ features are weaker than $f.z$, even if $f.x < f.z$ and $f.y < f.z$. Thus, for example, the minimal distinction between /p-b/ for the feature voicing will yield greater similarity than the /p-k/ pair, which is different by two place features, although voicing is a strong feature and place is a weak one. With the understanding that there are intra- and interfeature inequalities, it may be stated, then, that in spite of these inequalities, in general, the one-feature difference shows greater similarity or smaller difference than the two-feature difference, and the two-feature difference shows greater similarity or smaller distinction than the three-feature differences, and so on.

APPLICATION TO THERAPY: SAMPLE STRATEGIES, SIMILARITY COUNTS, AND COMPETENCE/PERFORMANCE

It will be demonstrated later that, in examining a child with articulation problems of the segmental type, it may be convenient to transfer his phonemic score to a distinctive feature score. When most of his problems are within the minimally distinct pairs, then it would be logical to find out what features are erred. Once the erred features are determined, a strategy of priority regarding the features should be established. Then, each time a feature needs to be worked with, the therapist must analyze the corpus of phonemes and determine whether he should start with the minus or the plus specifications of a given feature. This procedure applies to those children who have very minor articulation problems. For the child whose substitutions are among the double, triple, etc., distinct pairs, an entirely different strategy must be used. For example, if the majority of substitutions are between pairs with three-feature differences, the therapist should work systematically toward reducing them to two-feature errors, one-feature error, and then finally to no error. In such instances, one would have to proceed by working with the whole feature until the child finally has minimally distinct errors, after which work may be centered on the feature specification.

For example, assume that three children have substitution errors within the minimally distinct phoneme pairs. No child has errors within the nasal/non-nasal pairs, child 1 has some errors within the voiceless/voiced pairs, and children 2 and 3 have a number of errors within the place of articulation pairs. As has been described earlier, the nasality feature is more difficult to obliterate than the voicing feature, and the voicing feature is more difficult to obliterate than the place of articulation feature. On the basis of the hierarchy of the relative importance of the features—whose order in the present instance is: 1) nasality, 2) voicing, and 3) place of articulation—therapeutic work ought to begin with the voicing feature and proceed to the place of articulation feature since nasality was not in error. Because child 1 did not make all voicing errors that could have been made, it would be necessary to examine whether his voicing errors involved the minus or the plus specification of the feature. Assume that he has an error of plus specification (e.g., /p/ replaces /b/), then the corrective work ought to be initiated with such pairs alone. Because his substitutions, like those of the other two children, are all within the minimally distinct pairs, the place of articulation errors did not exist simultaneously with the voicing errors.

Assume also that an overall analysis of the children's substitution errors indicates that: 1) all their errors are within minimally distinct phoneme pairs, 2) the features already acquired are stronger (difficult to obliterate) than the ones not acquired, 3) the specifications of the acquired feature are systematic with the normal acquisition patterns, and 4) their competence reveals no errors. Competence may be described as the knowledge of the rules that generate phonological distinction. Usually, in phonological literature, competence is distinguished from performance. Performance is the actual realization (in the present instance it is the actual production of the phonemes) of the competence rules. It is assumed that competence precedes performance. In some instances a close examination of performance provides insight regarding competence of children.

In the above examples, child 1 has −voice/+voice substitutions, child 2 has place-2/place-3 substitutions, and child 3 has place-1/place-2 substitutions. According to the first child's system, he may be producing p/b, t/d, and k/g. According to the second child's system, he may be producing t/k and d/g, and according to the third child's system, he may be producing p/t and b/d (see Table 1-7).

The similarity count (or count of shared features) of the first child's system indicates that he has correctly realized place-1 in the p/b substitution, place-2 in the t/d substitution, and place-3 in the k/g substitution. Thus, his performance indicates that he has the competence or the correct knowledge of the place rules as realized in his substitutions. In each instance the place of articulation feature has been articulated correctly. But there definitely is a voicing error, and there is no indication that the child has competence of the feature

Table 1-7. Substitutions of three sample children

Child	Phoneme substitution	Target (erred) phoneme	Correct feature	Demonstration of competence/performance for correct feature
1	p/b	+Voice	Place-1	Competence
	t/d	+Voice	Place-2	Competence
	k/g	+Voice	Place-3	Competence
2	t/k	Place-3	−Voice	Competence
	d/g	Place-3	+Voice	Competence
3	p/t	Place-2	−Voice	Competence
	b/d	Place-2	+Voice	Competence

voicing. However, if one of the substitutions would have been p/d or t/g, then he would not have competence for either the voicing or the place feature.

The similarity count of the second child's system shows that, although the child has systematically erred place, voicing is realized correctly in the t/k and d/g substitutions. Thus, it seems that, competencewise, this child has no problems with the voicing feature.

The similarity count of the third child's system shows that, although the child has systematically erred place, his voicing is realized correctly in the p/t and b/d substitutions.

In examining a child's phoneme corpus, the therapist can ascertain from the substitutions the features that are absent and the features for which the child has competence. It is a much easier task in therapy when a child has competence for a feature but does not have performance than when both competence and performance for the feature are absent.

Table 1-8 shows that having competence of a feature and lacking performance (plus competence and minus performance) signifies a less serious problem than not having either competence or performance (minus competence and minus performance). When a speaker has both competence and performance (plus competence and plus performance) for a feature, he is normal. When he has performance without competence (plus performance and minus competence), which is rare, he has very serious problems. Imitation speech of severely mentally retarded patients may be placed in this last category.

SUMMARY

Thus far we have developed a series of interdependent procedures to evaluate the phonemic level on which a speaker operates. First, there is the utilization of phoneme, which serves as the foundation of the distinctive feature approach. In other words, the first thing to determine is the phonemic substitution. A distinctive feature matrix (where the consonants are presented in rows and the features in columns and where each consonant is specified at the intersection) is then utilized to unfold the phoneme substitution errors in terms of the distinctive features. The dissimilarity of the phonemes is described in a hierarchy of minimal, duple, triple, etc., distinctions that presupposes that a minimal distinction is a less severe substitution in speech production and perception than any other substitutions. A distinctive feature error may involve different specifications of a feature; i.e., a given specification may be more commonly erred than another. Finally, when both the similarity and the dissimilarity between the target and the substituted phoneme are considered along with the performance, the competence of the speaker regarding a feature is determined. The above step-by-step analysis of the substitutions of a speaker provides a comprehensive insight into the articulatory behavior of a speaker.

This chapter has dealt with the utilization of distinctive features for describing a set of only nine arbitrarily chosen English stop

Table 1-8. The four different possibilities of performance/competence combinations

	Competence	
Performance	(+)	(−)
(+)	No problem, e.g., normal speaker	Imitative speech only
(−)	Articulation problems	No speech

consonants. Only three features were utilized to explain them. Also, only the articulatory features were used. In actuality, the English language has 45 phonemes, which are traditionally described by different voicing, place, and manner features. In recent years (the last two decades) a number of feature systems have been developed. The next chapter deals with the description of the entire set of English consonants in terms of the different distinctive feature systems and the underlying basis of each.

chapter 2 Distinctive Feature Systems of Consonants

CONTENTS

Consonant feature systems
Jakobson, Fant, and Halle (1951)
Miller and Nicely (1955)
Halle (1964)
Singh and Black (1966)
Wickelgren (1966)
Chomsky and Halle (1968)
True perceptual feature system
Problems with feature systems
Multidimensional analysis
INDSCAL feature system proposed by Singh, Woods, and Becker

The consonant and vowel phonemes are coded by a series of distinctive features. The basis of these feature codes may be articulatory, perceptual, or acoustic. Usually, the consonants and vowels are coded separately because the production and perception of consonants and vowels have different bases. The production of vowels involves the periodic vibration of the vocal folds, and the production of consonants involves either no periodicity or quasiperiodicity only. Moreover, consonants are articulated with an obstruction somewhere in the vocal tract (mouth), and vowels are produced without (or with minimal) obstruction. For each consonant production, a constriction is created in the vocal tract because of the categorical contact of the articulators. Thus, for the production of the consonant /p/, the lips approximate categorically, while for the production of /f/ the lower lip and the upper teeth approximate. Vowels utilize the vocal tract as a resonator by altering the vocal tract configuration depending on the vowel being produced. For example, the production of the vowel /ɑ/ requires the maximal opening of the vocal tract whereas the production of the vowel /i/ requires only a minimal opening.

Also, there is evidence that the perception of vowels and the perception of consonants utilize differing strategies. Consonant perception is categorical, and thus utilizes the precise nature of the consonant production as reference, while vowel perception is continuous, implying that the vowel stimuli are perceived on an acoustic continuum. When competing consonants are presented to the left and right ears simultaneously, the consonant presented in the right ear is identified correctly a greater number of times than the consonant presented in the left ear (assuming that both ears have equal hearing thresholds). The conclusion is that consonant perception is lateralized in favor of the left hemisphere (right ear). The same experiment performed with pairs of vowels shows no such lateralization with any degree of clarity.

Because of the above basic important differences between vowels and consonants, vowels are rarely replaced by consonants and consonants are rarely replaced by vowels in articulation and identification. Vowels are substituted within the vowel category,and consonants are substituted within the consonant category. There are, however, some feature systems that describe vowels and consonants in terms of the same set of features. Even in these cases, it is seen clearly that the individual features of vowels and consonants do not apply to each other in any significant way; i.e., the vowel features (e.g., the feature rounding) do not generally describe the consonants, and the consonant features (e.g., the feature continuancy) do not describe the vowels (Chomsky and Halle, 1968, p. 176). The following section of this chapter deals with the consonant feature systems of English.

CONSONANT FEATURE SYSTEMS

Jakobson, Fant, and Halle (1951)

The pioneer work in the area of distinctive features was published by Jakobson, Fant, and Halle in 1951. The underlying basis of their work was the system of sounds, and the bulk of the evidence was presented in acoustic terms, mostly utilizing the spectrographic representation of sounds. Through spectrograms they were able to present a three-dimensional picture of the distinct pairs of consonants and vowels and demonstrate that clear acoustic distinctions exist between the minimally distinct pairs of phonemes. After examining the systematic acoustic distinctions of the phoneme pairs, they presented the articulatory basis of their acoustic findings. They examined a number of languages and found that the strategy of breaking the phoneme to its *ultimate unit,* i.e., distinctive feature, is universally applicable. The distinctive feature was considered the ultimate unit because it cannot be resolved any further into any finer unit of distinction.

Jakobson, Fant, and Halle concluded that "distinctive features which we detect in the languages of the world and which underlie their entire lexical and morphological stock amount to twelve binary oppositions: 1) vocalic/non-vocalic, 2) consonantal/non-consonantal, 3) interrupted/continuant, 4) checked/unchecked, 5) strident/mellow, 6) voiced/unvoiced, 7) compact/diffuse, 8) grave/acute, 9) flat/plain, 10) sharp/plain, 11) tense/lax, 12) nasal/oral" (p. 40). They further added that "no language contains all of these features" (p. 40). Only eight of these 12 features were used by them to describe 21 English consonants. Halle and Wickelgren used eight of the 12 features to describe 23 consonants of English. Jakobson, Fant, and Halle (1951, p. 43) proposed a feature system consisting of eight features on the basis of the Received Pronunciation (RP) of English.

Table 2-1 shows the eight features of the Jakobson, Fant, and Halle system, where a feature is denoted as tense/lax, nasal/oral, etc., depending on how the 21 consonants manifest these features. Also, Jakobson, Fant, and Halle specified the sounds of speech in terms of plus and minus specifications of the feature. The pluses indicate the presence of the first member of a feature, the minuses indicate the presence of the second member (or absence of the first member), and the blank spaces indicate the unimportance of both the first and second members in the description of that consonant. Thus, the first row signifies that the consonant /l/ has the presence of the vocalic feature and that all the other consonants have the absence of the vocalic feature. The second row indicates that the consonant /h/ has the absence of the consonantal feature. The third row indicates that /tʃ, dʒ, k, g, ʃ, ʒ, ŋ/ are compact consonants, /p, b, t, d, f, v, θ, ð, s, z, m, n/ are diffuse consonants, and the feature compact/diffuse is redundant for the consonants /l, h/, thus signifying the lack of relevance of this feature in describing these two consonants. A short description of each of the eight features of the Jakobson, Fant, and Halle system follows.

Vocalic/Nonvocalic The vowels of a language are considered as having the vocalic feature. The feature is marked by the "presence of the 'voice' source," which can be represented on a spectrogram by the clear formant characteristics in the lower one-third of the speech frequency region. Of the 21 English consonants included in the

Table 2-1. Jakobson, Fant, and Halle feature system for describing 21 English consonants

Feature	Consonant specification																				
	p	b	t	d	tʃ	dʒ	k	g	f	v	θ	ð	s	z	ʃ	ʒ	l	h	m	n	ŋ
Vocalic/nonvocalic	−	−	−	−	−	−	−	−	−	−	−	−	−	−	−	−	+	−	−	−	−
Consonantal/non-consonantal	+	+	+	+	+	+	+	+	+	+	+	+	+	+	+	+	+	−	+	+	+
Compact/diffuse	−	−	−	−	+	+	+	+	−	−	−	−	−	−	+	+			−	−	+
Grave/acute	+	+	−	−					+	+	−	−	−	−					+	−	
Nasal/oral	−	−	−	−	−	−	−	−	−	−	−	−	−	−	−	−			+	+	+
Tense/lax	+	−	+	−	+	−	+	−	+	−	+	−	+	−	+	−		+			
Continuant/interrupted	−	−	−	−	−	−	−	−	+	+	+	+	+	+	+	+					
Strident/mellow					+	+	−	−			−	−	+	+							

Jakobson, Fant, and Halle analysis, because all consonants except /l/ are considered to have the vocalic feature, the definition of the nonvocalic feature would imply the absence of all those specifications that were the attributes of the +vocalic feature.

Consonantal/Nonconsonantal The consonantal/nonconsonantal feature is the opposite of the vocalic/nonvocalic feature. Vocalic sounds are nonconsonantal, and nonvocalic sounds are consonantal. In other words, just as vocalic/nonvocalic distinctions primarily separate the vowels from the consonants, the consonantal/nonconsonantal feature also serves the same purpose. Only one consonant phoneme of English, /h/, has been marked nonconsonantal. Thus, except for /h/ all other consonants of English are consonantal, and except for /l/ all of the 21 consonants described here are nonvocalic. It is because of the sounds /h/ and /l/ that the features vocalic/nonvocalic and consonantal/nonconsonantal are included in the description of consonants. If there were no /h/ among the English consonants, then all 21 consonants would be consonantal, and therefore the need for that feature would not arise. Consistent with the classification of vocalic/nonvocalic feature, the consonantal/nonconsonantal feature is also considered a *fundamental source feature*.

Compact/Diffuse The basic distinction between the compact and diffuse features is in terms of the location of the energy in the frequency region of the speech sounds. Compactness is defined by the concentration of energy in one central frequency region, and diffuseness is described as the presence of one or more frequency concentrations in the noncentral (i.e., low or high or both) frequency regions. The consonants /tʃ, dʒ, k, g, ʃ, ʒ, ŋ/ are compact and the remaining consonants are diffuse, except /l, h/, for which the compact/diffuse feature is irrelevant.

The compact/diffuse feature has been labeled as a *resonance feature* because the compact consonants /tʃ, dʒ, k, g, ʃ, ʒ, ŋ/ are produced at the posterior part (palate and velum) of the vocal tract and the diffuse consonants are produced at the anterior part (lips, teeth, and alveolar ridge). In the case of compact consonants, the resonance is less behind the point of constriction of the oral cavity and more in front. On the other hand, the diffuse consonants have more resonance behind the point of constriction and less resonance in front. Actually, there is no resonating cavity in front of labial consonants. Articulatorily, the compact sounds are posterior (palatal or velar) and the diffuse consonants are anterior (labial, interdental, and alveolar).

Grave/Acute The grave/acute feature is explained with reference to the compact/diffuse feature because it relates only to diffuseness. Diffuse consonants with energy concentrated in the upper portion of the speech frequency region are considered acute. Diffuse consonants with energy concentrated in the lower portion of the speech frequency region are considered grave. Because compact consonants have frequency concentration only in the central region, they cannot be described in terms of gravity or acuteness and are considered redundant or irrelevant in reference to the grave/acute feature. Of the 21 English consonants, the consonants /p, b, f, v, m/ are grave consonants, the consonants /t, d, θ, ð, s, z, n/ are acute consonants, and the grave/acute feature is irrelevant for the consonants /tʃ, dʒ, k, g, ʃ, ʒ, ŋ, l, h/ (the first seven consonants being compact). Grave/acute is considered a *tonality feature* because the dichotomy between grave and acute mainly depends on the extreme frequencies (very low or very high) in the speech frequency regions.

Nasal/Oral The nasal consonants are described as having one narrow band of energy at a very low frequency (approximately 200 Hz) and another at a relatively high frequency (approximately 2,500 Hz). The consonants (m, n, ŋ) are specified as nasal and all other consonants except /l/ and /h/ as oral. The nasal/oral distinction is possible mainly because of the supplemental resonator cavity, i.e., the nasal cavity (the primary resonating cavity being the oral cavity). This feature, therefore, is also labeled the *supplemental resonator feature.*

Tense/Lax The tense consonants are described as having a longer duration than their lax counterparts. Additionally, in stops, tense consonants have greater strength of explosion than their lax counterparts. Thus, stops /p, t, k/ are tense consonants because they manifest greater force of explosion than do /b, d, g/, their lax counterparts. Also, duration is greater for /p, t, k/ than for /b, d, g/. The other tense consonants are /ʃ, tʃ, f, s, θ, h/. It may be inferred from the above that /ʃ/ manifests greater length or duration and is therefore tense as compared to /ʒ/, its lax counterpart; so also /tʃ, f, s, θ/ have greater length (and are therefore tense) than their lax counterparts /dʒ, v, z, ð/. The consonant /h/ does not have a lax counterpart. Similar to the grave/acute feature, the tense/lax feature is included under the general classification of the *tonality feature,* perhaps because the tense consonants tend to have higher frequency components than their lax counterparts.

Continuant/Interrupted The continuant/interrupted feature forms a part of the *secondary consonantal source feature,* which, according to Jakobson, Fant, and Halle, includes two types of features due to the primary source: (a) the envelope feature and (b) the stridency feature. The feature continuant/interrupted is considered an envelope feature because there is a smooth envelope of energy (or a smooth onset of energy) for continuant consonants and an abrupt envelope of energy for interrupted consonants. The term *secondary consonantal source feature* indicates that the source of the sound is at the point of contact within the vocal tract itself. The continuant consonants are /f, v, θ, ð, s, z, ʃ, ʒ/, and the interrupted consonants are /p, t, k, b, d, g, tʃ, dʒ/. The feature continuant/interrupted does not apply to the remaining five consonants /m, n, ŋ, l, h/. Articulatorily, all fricatives are continuants, and all oral stops (and affricates) are interrupted.

Strident/Mellow Sounds with irregular or random distribution of waveform are considered strident, and sounds with relatively more regular waveform distribution are considered mellow. For example, on the spectrogram, /s/, a strident phoneme, shows a random distribution of waveform, and /k/, a mellow phoneme, shows a distribution that is more regular. Only four consonants /tʃ, dʒ, s, z/ were considered strident in the original Jakobson, Fant, and Halle feature system, and four consonants /k, g, θ, ð/ were considered mellow. The remaining consonants were considered redundant. Strident/mellow is also a *secondary consonantal source feature* because the source of the production of turbulant noise is within the oral cavity itself.

Hierarchy of the Eight Features In Figure 2-1, the eight features of the Jakobson, Fant, and Halle system are utilized in the drawing of a tree diagram to demonstrate the existence of a feature hierarchy. Although the order in which the features are arranged may be altered somewhat, the difference between any two features still would be the same. How two sounds differ may be determined by examining the branchings of the features to which any two sounds belong. For example, /f/ is different from /θ/ because it is a grave sound and /θ/ is an acute sound. This distinction is made at the fourth level of the branching in Figure 2–1. Before the fourth level, /f/ and /θ/ are grouped together at the first level of branching as nonvocalic, at the second level as consonantal, and at the third level as diffuse. Thus, /f/ and /θ/ share the features nonvocalic, consonantal, and diffuse, but they do not share the feature grave/acute. After the fourth level, /f/ and /θ/ are not differentiated for the features continuant, tense, and oral, thus indicating that they are additionally similar with respect to the features continuant/interrupted, tense/lax, and nasal/oral. Both are continuant, tense, and oral consonants.

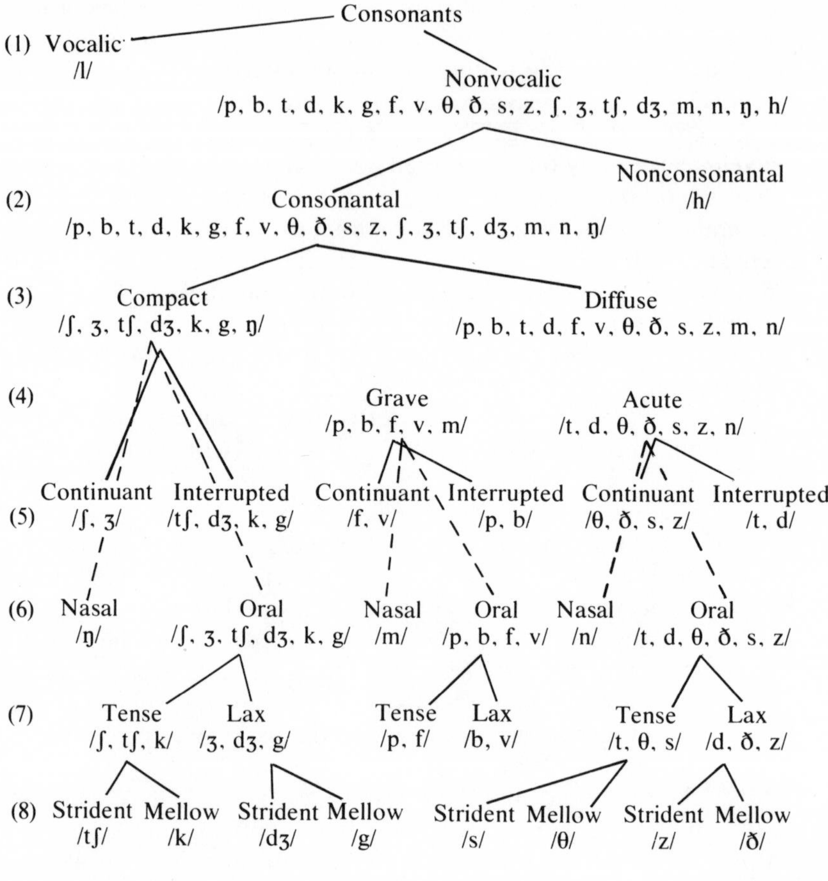

Figure 2-1. Representation of the Jakobson, Fant, and Halle feature system in a hierarchy of a tree diagram.

The basis of the Jakobson, Fant, and Halle system was the inspection of acoustic data pertaining to the phonemes of several languages. Once they were able to quantitatively discriminate one group of sounds, having one aspect of an acoustic feature, from another group of sounds, having the other aspect of that acoustic feature, they then inferred productive and perceptual correlates of the feature.

Miller and Nicely (1955)

Miller and Nicely (1955) described 16 consonants of English using a five-feature system consisting of voicing, duration, affrication, place, and nasality. Unlike Jakobson, Fant, and Halle, who described 21 consonants in terms of eight acoustic features, Miller and Nicely described 16 consonants in terms of four articulatory and one acoustic feature. The articulatory features were voicing, affrication, place, and nasality, and the acoustic feature was duration. Unlike Jakobson, Fant, and Halle, Miller and Nicely denoted each consonant by the presence or absence of a feature. They did not leave any consonant unspecified in terms of either having or not having a feature. They disregarded this concept of phonological redundancy of a feature for a group of consonants. They relied heavily on the actual phonetic elements of the consonants.

Miller and Nicely designated 1 to a consonant having a feature and 0 to a consonant not having a feature. The basis of their feature system was the inspection of 17 different "confusion matrices" (a term first used by Miller and Nicely) resulting from listening to the 16 consonants in the context of monosyllabic /a/ under five different levels of noise and 11 different bands of frequencies. A confusion matrix is a matrix with sounds used as stimuli at the extreme left of the rows and sounds used as responses at the head of the columns; the entries at the intersection of the stimuli and responses represent the number of times the stimulus has been confused with the response. The basis of their feature system was the errors (confusions) made by listeners in identifying the 16 different consonants. Noise and high and low bandpass filtering distortions were introduced to elicit errors from listeners. Once the errors were elicited, Miller and Nicely grouped the consonants according to the tendencies in clustering of the errors. For example, in most cases stops were misperceived as other stops (e.g., /t/ was perceived as /p/) while fricatives were misperceived as other fricatives (e.g., /θ/ was perceived as /f/). Such distribution of errors provided insight for proposing the feature "affricate," which separated stops from fricatives. Miller and Nicely examined other clustering of errors in all of the 17 confusion matrices. For example, the feature nasality was proposed because nasal consonants tended to be erred as nasals and non-nasal consonants tended to be erred as non-nasals. A similar trend was found for the features voicing, duration, and place of articulation.

The Miller and Nicely feature system represents a significant departure from the Jakobson, Fant, and Halle feature system.

Whereas all features in the Jakobson, Fant, and Halle system were binary, Miller and Nicely proposed a ternary feature: place of articulation. Also, instead of specifying the presence of a feature by plus, the absence by minus, and redundancy by leaving a blank, Miller and Nicely specified the presence of a feature by 1 and the absence by 0 (Table 2-2). There was no blank, presumably because they considered that neither phonological nor acoustic redundancy applied to the perception of these consonants.

The feature system proposed by Miller and Nicely was a perceptual feature system. The basis for choosing the features and their given specifications was somewhat arbitrary. However, when they utilized their feature system to predict the confusions of the 16 English consonants, their results were promising.

In addition, they used more conventional terminology to code the 16 English consonants used in their experiments. They eliminated the complexity of Jakobson, Fant, and Halle's labeling of the features by: 1) not listing both members of a feature, e.g., voiced/unvoiced, nasal/oral, etc., and 2) using the term "voicing," which implied both plus and minus specifications of the features. The +voicing was denoted by 1 and the −voicing by 0. Miller and Nicely proposed a perceptual feature system although the references of the features were predominately articulatory.

Voicing In the Miller and Nicely feature matrix, the feature voicing is differentiated as voiced or voiceless, where voiced is designated by 1 and voiceless by 0. The voiced consonants are produced with vibrations of the vocal folds. The voiceless consonants are produced without vibration of the vocal folds. Thus, the voiceless consonants, in acoustic terms, are more noisy than the voiced. The consonants /b, g, d, v, ð, z, ʒ, m, n/ are voiced and /p, t, k, f, θ, s, ʃ/ are voiceless.

Duration Duration is primarily an acoustic feature. Miller and Nicely were the first to suggest the importance of acoustic characteristics of some fricative consonants in perception. The consonants with a greater amount of duration than the other fricative consonants are /s, z, ʃ, ʒ/. These four consonants decidedly have greater duration than the rest of the 16 consonants and, in Miller and Nicely's opinion, it is their extra duration that is the most effective in setting them apart.

Affrication If the closure at the point of contact between the articulator and the point of articulation is complete, the consonant may be either a stop or a nasal, but if the closure is such that at the

Table 2-2. Miller and Nicely feature system

Feature	Consonant specification															
	p	t	k	f	θ	s	ʃ	b	d	g	v	ð	z	ʒ	m	n
Voicing	0	0	0	0	0	0	0	1	1	1	1	1	1	1	1	1
Duration	0	0	0	0	0	1	1	0	0	0	0	0	1	1	0	0
Affrication	0	0	0	1	1	1	1	0	0	0	1	1	1	1	0	0
Place	0	1	2	0	1	1	2	0	1	2	0	1	1	2	0	1
Nasality	0	0	0	0	0	0	0	0	0	0	0	0	0	0	1	1

point of contact air is forced through a narrow aperture (in the shape of a slit or a groove) the result is a kind of turbulence or a friction noise that distinguishes /f, θ, s, ʃ, v, ð, z, ʒ/ from /p, t, k, b, d, g, m, n/ among the 16 consonants included in the Miller and Nicely experiment.

Place of Articulation The three different specifications for the place of articulation feature are front, mid, and back depending on the area in the mouth where the constriction is formed. If the constriction is in the front of the mouth, the designation is place-0; the consonants that are designated place-0 are /p, b, f, v, m/. A constriction in the middle of the mouth is considered place-1; the consonants that are designated place-1 are /t, d, θ, ð, s, z, n/. Finally, a constriction in the back of the mouth is considered place-2; the consonants that are designated place-2 are /ʃ, ʒ, k, g/.

It may be pointed out that assignment of the numbers 0, 1, and 2 for the front, mid, and back consonants, respectively, is arbitrary. It would have been equally logical to label the back consonants as place-0, mid consonants as place-1, and front consonants as place-2. As long as the basic assumption—that back is closer to mid than it is to front and that front is closer to mid than it is to back—is not invalidated, any assignment of value to front, mid, and back places on a continuum will not alter their interrelationships in terms of place of articulation. For example, let the front, mid, and back places have 0, 1, and 2 values, respectively, in one instance and 2, 1, and 0 values, respectively, in another. The ultimate result when describing differences between phonemes is the same. In the event that front is place-0, mid is place-1, and back is place-2, the difference between front and mid is one ($1 - 0 = 1$), between front and back is two ($2 - 0 = 2$), and between mid and back is one ($2 - 1 = 1$). In the event that front is place-2, mid is place-1, and back is place-0, the difference between front and mid is again one ($2 - 1 = 1$), between front and back is two ($2 - 0 = 2$), and between mid and back is one ($1 - 0 = 1$).

Nasality The nasal consonants are produced by opening the nasopharyngeal port and releasing the intraoral air pressure through the nose. The consonants /m, n/ are nasals and the remaining 14 consonants are non-nasals.

Halle (1964)

Utilizing the features proposed by Jakobson, Fant, and Halle, Halle (1964) described 18 consonants of English. However, some crucial differences exist between the two feature systems. Halle designated plus or minus to each consonant, thus doing away with the idea of designating redundancy by leaving a blank. Also, instead of naming a feature by both of its opposing members, e.g., vocalic/nonvocalic, he utilized only one of the two aspects of a feature, e.g., vocalic, assuming that the plus specification would indicate the presence and the minus specification would indicate the absence of a feature. Additionally, the articulatory descriptions of the distinctive features, what he called the "articulatory correlates of the distinctive features," became a prominent and sole basis for his feature system. Note, however, that in a footnote of the chapter he maintains his allegiance to the acoustic correlates of the distinctive features as proposed originally by Jakobson, Fant, and Halle. He writes: "The fact that in the following list, reference is made only to the articulatory properties of speech and nothing is said about the acoustical properties, is not to be taken as an indication that the latter are somewhat less important. The only reason for concentrating here exclusively on the former is that these are more readily observed without instruments." Table 2-3 summarizes the eight features that Halle used to describe 18 English consonants.

Vocalic The periodic excitation of the vocal folds and the openness of the vocal tract form the articulatory correlates of vocalic sounds. The nonvocalic sounds, however, are produced with no periodic excitation of the vocal folds and with a narrow opening of the vocal tract. In traditional articulatory terms, it could be said that, generally, vowels are vocalic and consonants are nonvocalic.

Consonantal In the Halle feature system, all 18 consonants are labeled −vocalic and +consonantal. Because the Halle feature system consists of 18 consonants, all of which are −vocalic and +consonantal, these two features do not distinguish any one consonant from the other and, therefore, are not necessary for their set. Halle describes consonants as those sounds produced with *occlusion* or *contact* in the center path through the oral cavity, and nonconsonantal sounds as those produced without the occlusion. A maximal amount of occlusion of the oral cavity produces stops /p, t, k, b, d, g, m, n/. A relatively less amount of occlusion produces fricatives /f, v, θ, ð, s, z, ʃ, ʒ/. A still lesser degree of occlusion would produce "vowel-like" consonants /j, r, l, w/ if Halle had extended his system to include them. Finally, the least amount of occlusion in the oral cavity produces the vowel sounds. Most consonantal sounds belong to one of the first three levels of occlusions: 1) maximal occlusion = stops, 2) second degree of occlusion = fricatives, and 3) third degree of occlusion = liquids and glides.

Table 2-3. Halle feature system describing 18 English consonants

Feature	Consonant specification																	
	p	b	m	f	v	k	g	t	d	θ	ð	n	s	z	tʃ	dʒ	ʃ	ʒ
Vocalic	–	–	–	–	–	–	–	–	–	–	–	–	–	–	–	–	–	–
Consonantal	+	+	+	+	+	+	+	+	+	+	+	+	+	+	+	+	+	+
Grave	+	+	+	+	+	–	–	–	–	–	–	–	–	–	–	–	–	–
Diffuse	+	+	+	+	+	–	–	+	+	+	+	+	+	+	–	–	–	–
Strident	–	–	–	+	+	–	–	–	–	–	–	–	+	+	+	+	+	+
Nasal	–	–	+	–	–	–	–	–	–	–	–	+	–	–	–	–	–	–
Continuant	–	–	–	+	+	–	–	–	–	+	+	–	+	+	–	–	+	+
Voiced	–	+	+	–	+	–	+	–	+	–	+	+	–	+	–	+	–	+

Grave The definition of grave in this system is the same as that in the Jakobson, Fant, and Halle feature system. Thus, Halle considers /p, b, f, v, m/ as grave and /t, d, θ, ð, n, s, z, tʃ, dʒ, ʃ, ʒ, k, g/ as acute sounds.

Diffuse The diffuseness feature is designated to consonants, and the feature compactness is designated solely to vowels. Thus, consonants are characterized as diffuse/nondiffuse in the Halle system, rather than compact/diffuse as in the Jakobson, Fant, and Halle system. Diffuse sounds are located in the anterior portion of the vocal tract and are produced with the utmost narrowing of the air passage in the vocal tract. They are /p, b, m, f, v, t, d, θ, ð, n, s, z/. The remaining consonants /k, g, tʃ, dʒ, ʃ, ʒ/ are nondiffuse sounds. It may be noted that, from the point of view of articulatory positions, diffuse consonants are labials, labiodentals, interdentals, and alveolars. The nondiffuse consonants are produced at the posterior portion of the mouth with lesser degree of the narrowing of the air passage in the vocal tract. From the point of view of articulatory positions, these consonants are velars /k, g/ and palatals /tʃ, dʒ, ʃ, ʒ/.

Strident The strident consonants are produced by friction of the air stream directed across a sharp-edge constriction in the vocal tract. The main characteristic of the stridency feature is the maximal emission of noise produced by the friction created by the air stream emitted across the constriction. Halle considers /f, v, s, z, ʃ, ʒ, tʃ, dʒ/ as strident consonants and the remaining 12 consonants as nonstrident. It may be pointed out that six of these strident consonants /f, v, s, z, ʃ, ʒ/ are fricatives and two /tʃ, dʒ/ are affricates (the fricatives not considered strident are /θ, ð, h/).

Nasal Nasal consonants are produced by the lowering of the velum, thereby passing the air through the nasal cavity, whereas oral consonants are produced by the raising of the velum, thereby releasing the air through the oral cavity. The consonants /m, n/ are nasal and the remaining consonants are non-nasal.

Continuant The continuant sounds are produced by the narrowing of the vocal tract in such a fashion that the narrowing phenomenon does not cause total occlusion. The noncontinuant sounds, on the other hand, are totally occluded at some point in the vocal tract. The noncontinuant sounds, which involve complete closure at the point of articulation in the vocal tract, are /p, b, m, k, g, t, d, n, tʃ, dʒ/. The continuant sounds, which involve a relatively free flow of air from the glottis to the lips, are /f, v, θ, ð, s, z, ʃ, ʒ/.

Voiced Production of the voiced sounds involves the vibration of the vocal folds, and production of the voiceless sounds involves no vibration of the vocal folds. Thus, /p, t, k, f, θ, s, ʃ, tʃ/ are voiceless consonants and /b, d, g, v, ð, z, ʒ, dʒ, m, n/ are voiced consonants.

Application of Halle's System At the basis of Halle's proposal of a distinctive feature system is the following theory: Given that there is a small set of universal attributes that describe the phonetic properties of all languages of the world, it would appear that these attributes are innate and not a product of cultural backgrounds. The research in different areas of the application of distinctive features to phoneme production and perception has substantiated Halle's claim that features or "attributes" are indeed related to "something fairly basic in man's constitution." In Chapters 5 and 6, the perceptual correlates of the distinctive features of consonants and vowels will be reported, and they substantiate the above hypothesis. The actual number of these universal features has changed between the years 1951 (Jakobson, Fant, and Halle) and 1972 (Stevens and House). Jakobson, Fant, and Halle originally proposed 12 features for coding all phonemes in all languages of the world. Halle revised this in 1964, proposing 15 features. In a recent (1972) article, Stevens and House claim that between 25 and 30 features are needed to account for the coding of phonemes in all languages.

From the research cited above, speech pathologists and audiologists need not inherit the theoretical disagreement regarding how many features are needed to account for all the phonemic systems of the languages of the world. What is more important to them is the knowledge that phonemes are coded by distinctive features and that distinctive features are basic attributes of phonemes related closely to the human response system. It would be logical, then, to tap these features as tools for evaluative and corrective purposes when the problems of phoneme production and/or perception are involved.

Singh and Black (1966)

Singh and Black (1966) extended the Miller and Nicely feature system by adding: 1) liquid, to distinguish /b/ from /w/ and /g/ from /j/, 2) retroflexion, to distinguish /r/ from /l/, and 3) a fourth value to the place feature, to distinguish /tʃ/ from /h/. This feature system is considered an extension simply because Singh and Black utilized the features voicing, duration, affrication, and nasality without altering the way in which Miller and Nicely had used them. The two additional features and an additional specification of the place feature were necessary to distinguish the 21 English phonemes from each other.

Because Miller and Nicely used only 16 consonants and most of them formed groups of natural classes, a limited number of features was needed to specify them. Singh and Black used 26 consonants, of which 21 belonged to English and five belonged to three other languages from which they had drawn their speakers and listeners.

The confusion matrices in the Singh and Black study depended on the differing degree of linguistic familiarity of the test consonants. Native speakers and listeners of English, Hindi, Japanese, and Arabic produced and identified the 26 consonants, the majority of which belonged to English. Because the source of error was present in both speaking and listening of the native and foreign sounds, the errors of both the speakers and listeners of the four languages were analyzed. Subjects speaking the consonants of a foreign language were expected to make greater productive errors than the subjects speaking their native language. Also, the subjects listening to the sounds of a foreign language were expected to make greater perceptual errors than the subjects listening to the sounds of their own language. The focal point was to consider cross-linguistic errors that were somewhat similar to the patterns of errors (or confusions) generated by the noise and filtering conditions in the Miller and Nicely (1955) experiment. The assumption was that, no matter what the source of the error, it will be accounted for by the distinctive features of the phoneme. Consistent with the earlier proposed hypothesis that distinctive features trigger some innate human response to phonemes and that this innateness is common to all men (irrespective of their own linguistic backgrounds), the speakers and listeners of the four languages were utilized to test the hypothesis of a universal treatment of features across four languages.

Table 2-4 shows how the six features of the Singh and Black system are designated to the 21 consonants of English. The feature aspiration, which is phonemic in Hindi and Arabic languages, was the seventh feature in the Singh and Black system. Aspiration is not included in the table because this feature system is presented here in the context of English consonants.

Voicing The nine consonants /p, t, k, s, ʃ, h, tʃ, f, θ/ are voiceless; the remaining 12 consonants are voiced.

Nasality The two sounds /m, n/ are nasal, and the remaining 19 sounds are non-nasal.

Frication The 11 consonants /f, v, θ, ð, s, z, ʃ, ʒ, tʃ, dʒ, h/ are classified as fricative, and the remaining 10 are classified as non-fricative.

Table 2-4. Singh and Black (1966) feature system

	Consonant specification																				
Feature	p	b	t	d	k	g	s	z	ʃ	ʒ	f	v	θ	ð	h	tʃ	dʒ	l	r	m	n
Voicing	0	1	0	1	0	1	0	1	0	1	0	1	0	1	0	0	1	1	1	1	1
Nasality	0	0	0	0	0	0	0	0	0	0	0	0	0	0	0	0	0	0	0	1	1
Frication	0	0	0	0	0	0	1	1	1	1	1	1	1	1	1	1	1	0	0	0	0
Place	1	1	2	2	4	4	2	2	3	3	1	1	2	2	4	3	3	2	3	1	2
Duration	0	0	0	0	0	0	1	1	1	1	0	0	0	0	0	0	0	0	0	0	0
Liquid	0	0	0	0	0	0	0	0	0	0	0	0	0	0	0	0	0	1	1	0	0

Place of Articulation The place of articulation is a quaternary feature in which four places are specified: 1) front of the mouth /p, f, b, v, m/, 2) mid-front of the mouth /t, d, s, z, θ, ð, l, n/, 3) mid-back of the mouth /ʃ, ʒ, tʃ, dʒ, r/, and 4) back of the mouth /k, g, h/. In order to avoid a great deal of overlap, the place of articulation feature was not considered binary. Instead, it was described as a multiple channel system consisting of the four places described above. Another option is to treat the place of articulation feature as having four separate channels: 1) labial/nonlabial, 2) alveolar/nonalveolar, 3) palatal/non-palatal, and 4) velar/nonvelar. However, it has been shown (Singh, 1966) that the multiple channel system is not only economical but increases the efficiency of the system and is equally valid. Therefore, instead of defining the phoneme /k/ in terms of the four separate channels as being nonlabial, nonalveolar, and nonpalatal, it is defined in terms of the multiple channel system as being place-4 (back of the mouth), which describes precisely that /k/ is not place-1, place-2, or place-3. Similarly, /tʃ/ is defined as being place-3, /t/ as place-2, and /p/ as place-1.

Duration Four sounds are classified as having a long duration /s, z, ʃ, ʒ/; the remaining 17 sounds are classified as being relatively shorter.

Liquid The consonant /l/ is considered a liquid and the remaining 20 consonants are nonliquid.

Extension of Singh and Black System The Singh and Black feature system was further extended in another study (Singh, 1968) to include all the consonants of English. In addition to the six features discussed above, Singh (1968) added the feature glide to distinguish /w/, /j/, and /m/ from the rest of the consonants of English, and the feature retroflex to distinguish /r/ from the rest of the consonants of English. The feature system proposed by Singh included eight features, of which seven were binary—namely, voicing, nasality, frication, duration, liquid, glide, and retroflex—and one was quaternary, namely, the place of articulation feature. The Singh feature system is a completed feature system because it distinguishes all the 25 consonants of English from one another.

The Singh (1968) system was devised to interpret the perceptual errors of Multiple Choice Intelligibility Tests. A Multiple Choice Intelligibility Test requires a listener to identify a word from a group of four similar sounding words (one stimulus word and three decoy words). The stimulus word and the three decoy words appear together on the listener's response sheet. It was found that the stimulus word was most frequently identified (as itself), but when it was identified incorrectly the chosen error depended on the number of distinctive feature differences between the stimulus word and the error response. This distinctive feature disparity was computed with the help of Table 2-5. The computed results indicating the degree of similarity of distinctive features are a reliable predictor of the relative order of preference of listeners' responses. These findings were true in the context of one- and two-syllable meaningful words and nonsense syllables, in closed and open-choice tests, and in various signal-to-noise, filter, and speaking-listening group conditions.

Wickelgren (1966)

Wickelgren (1966) noted that, in short-term memory tasks, when subjects recall consecutive consonants, the intruded consonants are related to the stimulus phoneme. This relationship between the intended and intruded phonemes was predicted significantly by several distinctive feature systems including the one proposed by Wickelgren. The hypothesis was that if the intended phoneme and the intruded phoneme share a majority of features, and if they always seem to differ by one or two features, it may be concluded that the phoneme coding takes place in terms of the distinctive features.

Wickelgren listed two purposes for conducting his experiment: 1) to determine if errors in short-term memory for consonants tend to have features in common with the correct consonant, and 2) to determine what distinctive feature system best predicts these errors. It may be recalled that Wickelgren had at his disposal the Jakobson, Fant, and Halle feature system to compare relative efficacies in the prediction of the errors in short-term memory. Wickelgren chose to utilize the Miller and Nicely and the Halle feature systems. He easily converted from Halle's system the plus to one and the minus to zero, thereby establishing an equitable basis for comparing the Miller and Nicely and the Halle feature systems.

Wickelgren also proposed his own feature system as a result of inspecting the clustering patterns of the matrices of consonant errors generated in his short-term memory experiments. Although he was satisfied with the Miller and Nicely feature system, he knew that, if Miller and Nicely's system were to be extended to his 22 English consonants, it would require some additional dimensions or values to handle laterals, semivowels, and the consonants /t/, /d/, and /h/. Wickelgren had one of two courses to adopt to handle the above consonants: 1) to extend the Miller and Nicely feature system, accept-

Table 2-5. Singh feature system to describe all English consonants

	Consonant specification																							
Feature	p	b	m	t	d	n	tʃ	dʒ	k	g	f	v	θ	ð	s	z	ʃ	ʒ	w	r	l	j	h	ŋ	ʍ
Voicing	0	1	1	0	1	1	0	1	0	1	0	1	0	1	0	1	0	1	1	1	1	1	0	1	0
Nasality	0	0	1	0	0	1	0	0	0	0	0	0	0	0	0	0	0	0	0	0	0	0	0	1	0
Frication	0	0	0	0	0	0	1	1	0	0	1	1	1	1	1	1	1	1	0	0	0	0	1	0	1
Duration	0	0	0	0	0	0	0	0	0	0	0	0	0	0	1	1	1	1	0	0	0	0	0	0	0
Liquid	0	0	0	0	0	0	0	0	0	0	0	0	0	0	0	0	0	0	0	1	1	0	0	0	0
Glide	0	0	0	0	0	0	0	0	0	0	0	0	0	0	0	0	0	0	1	0	0	1	0	0	1
Retroflex	0	0	0	0	0	0	0	0	0	0	0	0	0	0	0	0	0	0	0	1	0	0	0	0	0
Place	1	1	1	2	2	2	3	3	4	4	1	1	2	2	2	2	3	3	1	2	2	3	4	4	1

ing their basic classifications (as Singh and Black did), or 2) to accept some of the Miller and Nicely classifications and to introduce some new ones, still in keeping with the articulatory hypothesis of Miller and Nicely. Wickelgren adopted the second course. He proposed a new feature system, now shown as the Wickelgren feature system. Another reason for proposing a new feature system was his theoretical disagreement with the Halle feature system. Even before Wickelgren had found that the Halle feature system showed poor predictability in short-term memory, he was skeptical about the feature system. Here is how he reflected on the Halle feature system (Wickelgren, 1966, p. 389):

> Halle has eight binary dimensions on which consonants are classified. The rather large number of dimensions result from the decision to use only two values per dimension. Halle gives a moderately complicated articulatory description of the value of the dimensions in the Halle system, but the system is unnatural and inelegant as a description of articulation and no attempt is made by Halle to validate the system on these grounds.

Wickelgren's efforts to propose a natural and elegant feature system enabled him to: 1) retain Miller and Nicely's nasality and voicing features, 2) make finer distinction on the place continuum, thus increasing Miller and Nicely's three places to five, and most importantly 3) introduce a new approach to handle the manner of articulation. The approach allowed room for handling (at least theoretically) stops, fricatives, sonorants (vowel-like consonants), and vowels on a continuum, the continuum being named "openness." Naturally, the stops are considered as having the least degree of openness, fricatives as having the second degree of openness, and vowel-like sounds as having the third degree of openness of the vocal tract. The Wickelgren system has two binary features (voicing and nasality), one ternary feature (openness), and one feature with five specifications. Actually, if the Wickelgren feature system were strictly binary and if he had utilized all the parameters that he believed constituted the consonants, then his feature system would contain 10 features: 1) voiced/voiceless, 2) nasal/non-nasal, 3) first degree of openness/absence of first degree of openness, 4) second degree of openness/absence of second degree of openness, 5) third degree of openness/absence of third degree of openness, 6) place-1/absence of place-1, 7) place-2/absence of place-2, 8) place-3/absence of place-3, 9) place-4/absence of place-4, and 10) place-5/absence of place-5.

Obviously, this would be a very inelegant feature system because there would be a large amount of overlap among the three minus openness specifications and the five minus place feature specifications.

Table 2-6 describes the four-feature system devised by Wickelgren. The features voicing and nasality are the same as those described in the Miller and Nicely and the Singh and Black feature systems. Wickelgren's introduction to a 5 specification of the place feature divided the 22 consonants into the following groups: place-0 /p, b, m, f, w, v/, place-1 /t, d, n, θ, ð, r/, place-2 /s, z, l/, place-3 /tʃ, dʒ, ʃ, j/, and place-4 /k, g, h/. The three specifications of the feature openness divided the 22 consonants into the following groups: zero degree of openness /p, b, m, t, d, n, tʃ, dʒ, k, g/, one degree of openness /f, v, θ, ð, s, z, ʃ/, and two degrees of openness /w, r, l, j, h/.

Wickelgren considered openness as a common feature in describing the consonants and vowels on a single continuum. He wrote: "Notice that the openness of the vocal tract and place of articulation are the same two dimensions that were so accurate in predicting the errors in STM [short-term memory] for English vowels. Of course, the values of the openness dimensions for vowels would begin with a value greater than that for the semivowels. Thus, openness is conceived to code on a single 6-point scale the difference between (1) stop consonants; (2) fricatives; (3) semivowels, laterals, and /h/; (4) high (narrow-opening) vowels; (5) medium vowels, and (6) low (wide-opening) vowels. Values of the place dimensions for vowels lie within the range for consonants."

Chomsky and Halle (1968)

Chomsky and Halle (1968) provided elaborate phonological grounds (data) for extracting a set of articulatory distinctive features. According to Chomsky and Halle, the phonological components form a system of rules that relate to the phonetic representation of the sounds of a language. Chomsky and Halle extracted distinctive features by examining different hierarchies of the linguistic rules. For example, a sentence in a language is generated by syntactic rules that determine the sequencing of phrases and the classes of words within the phrases. The words in turn consist of sequences of phonemes. The phonemes can be represented by a feature matrix in which the rows correspond to a restricted set of universal phonetic categories and the columns correspond to phonemes. A sentence, *The boy hit the ball,*

Table 2-6. Wickelgren feature system

	Consonant specification																					
Feature	p	b	t	d	tʃ	dʒ	k	g	f	v	θ	ð	s	z	ʃ	w	r	l	j	h	m	n
Voicing	0	1	0	1	0	1	0	1	0	1	0	1	0	1	0	1	1	1	1	0	1	1
Nasality	0	0	0	0	0	0	0	0	0	0	0	0	0	0	0	0	0	0	0	0	1	1
Openness	1	1	1	1	1	1	1	1	2	2	2	2	2	2	2	3	3	3	3	3	1	1
Place	1	1	2	2	4	4	5	5	1	1	2	2	3	3	4	1	2	3	4	5	1	2

may be described hierarchically, first by the syntactic rules, then by the lexical rule, then by the phonemic sequencing rule, and lastly by the distinctive feature rule.

Chomsky and Halle described the articulatory features of the universal sounds on the assumption that the configurations of the human vocal mechanism and the speech reception mechanism are identical for all men. They mapped out the vocal mechanisms in terms of the source of sound, the different areas of the vocal tract involved, and the different positions of the tongue in relation to the different areas of the vocal tract. They also took into account the nasal/oral cavity differences that relate to the nasal/oral sounds. They felt an urgent need for a universal set of parameters that could be commonly utilized to describe the sounds of all the languages of the world. These features are based on the phonetic or the articulatory possibilities of man. Each feature is binary and is defined by antonymous adjectives: voiced/nonvoiced (voiceless), nasal/non-nasal (oral), vocalic/non-vocalic, etc.

For the student of English phonetics, it would not be necessary to describe all the articulatory features that represent the phonetic capabilities of all men. Obviously, no one language utilizes all those features. However, for a student of articulation disorders, such an inventory may be extremely valuable. If a speaker is substituting strictly within the phonological realm of the English language, his errors are commonly labeled as substitution errors, and the speech therapist only has to work with the features that describe English sounds. However, if a speaker is substituting outside of the realm of the English language, his errors are described as distortion errors. Since the Chomsky-Halle inventory includes all that the human articulators are capable of producing, a thorough understanding of these features might be useful for a speech therapist in unfolding systematically the mysteries of speech sound distortions.

There are five major categories in the universal phonetic features of the Chomsky and Halle feature system. They are: 1) major class features, 2) cavity features, 3) manner of articulation features, 4) source features, and 5) prosodic features.

Major Class Features Major class features divide the broad phonetic categories into: 1) true consonants (consonantal), 2) vowels (vocalic), and 3) consonants that have a vowel-like nature (sonorant). These features relate to the closing/opening phenomena of the vocal tract. According to Chomsky and Halle: "During the closed phase the flow of air from the lungs is either impeded or stopped, and pressure is built up in the vocal tract; during the open phase, air flows out freely'' (1968, pp. 301–302).

Consonantal/Nonconsonantal The consonantal sounds are produced with obstruction somewhere in the vocal tract, and the nonconsonantal sounds are produced without such obstruction. All English vowels, glides, and the consonant /h/ are considered nonconsonantal because their production does not involve any obstruction in the midsagittal region of the vocal tract.

Vocalic/Nonvocalic Vocalic sounds are produced only when the most radical constriction in the oral cavity does not exceed that in the vowels /i/ and /u/, and when the vocal cords are positioned to produce ''spontaneous voicing.'' It may be pointed out that /i/ and /u/ are the most constricted of all vowels in English. Thus, by rule, any sound that is more constricted than /i/ and /u/ is nonvocalic; most of the nonvocalic sounds, therefore, are consonants. All English vowels and the liquid /l/ are vocalic sounds, and the remainder are nonvocalic sounds.

Sonorant/Nonsonorant Sonorants are produced with ''spontaneous voicing.'' Thus, any production of speech sound that does not involve spontaneous voicing is a nonsonorant sound. All voiceless consonants of English and all voiced consonants that are not glides, nasals, and liquids are nonsonorant. Sonorants include vowels, glides, nasals, and liquids of English. The sonorant consonants in English include glides /w, j/, nasals /m, n, ŋ/, and liquids /l, r/.

Cavity Features Cavity features are the second set of universal features described by Chomsky and Halle. Before describing the cavity features, Chomsky and Halle pointed out the problem with the International Phonetic Alphabet, in which the vowels and consonants are described by two different systems. The vowels are described by the location of the three general areas: front, mid, and back, and the consonants are described by the point of constriction in the oral cavity: labial, alveolar, etc. Jakobson's solution to these separate systems for vowels and consonants was the presentation of two sets of binary features: 1) compact/diffuse, and 2) grave/acute, which provided a unitary system for the descriptions of both vowels and consonants. Chomsky and Halle considered this unitary system (''in retrospect'') ''too radical a solution'' to the International Phonetic Alphabet dichotomy. The changes they suggested involve changes in terminology. They replaced the terms ''compact, diffuse, and grave'' by new terms.

The subclassifications of the cavity features are: 1) coronal, 2) anterior, 3) tongue body features: high, low, and back, 4) round, 5) distributed, 6) covered, 7) glottal constrictions, and 8) secondary apertures: nasal and lateral. It may be mentioned again that all these specifications of the cavity features are not normally used in the English language and that later on in this chapter a short description of only those features that are relevant to English is presented.

Coronal/Noncoronal Coronal in the Webster's *Third New International Dictionary* (1967) means retroflex, which in turn is described as "articulation with or involving the participation of the tongue tip curled up and back until its under surface touches the hard palate—used esp. of various consonants in Asiatic-Indian languages . . . *of a vowel:* articulated with or involving the participation of the tongue tip raised and retracted toward the hard palate." Chomsky and Halle described coronal sounds as produced with the blade of the tongue raised from its neutral position, and noncoronal sounds as produced with the blade of the tongue in the neutral position. Thus, although the traditional description of the term "coronal" may involve the tip of the tongue, Chomsky and Halle have attributed the feature to the phenomenon of tongue blade raising versus tongue blade neutral. It may be pointed out also that these authors "differed somewhat" in their definition of the terms from their source references (Sievers, 1901; Broch, 1911). Chomsky and Halle regarded as coronal all types of sounds formed with the blade of the tongue, but Sievers and Broch did not use this term when speaking of sounds formed with the flat part of the blade (Chomsky and Halle, 1968, p. 304).

The English consonants /r, l, t, d, θ, ð, n, s, z, tʃ, dʒ, ʃ, ʒ/ are considered as coronal and the remainder as noncoronal. In other words, according to Chomsky and Halle, the consonants listed above are coronal because they are all produced with the raised blade of the tongue. The noncoronal consonants such as /p, b, f, v, m, k, g, ŋ, h/ are produced with the neutral status of the tongue blade. Actually, the first five of the nine noncoronal consonants do not involve the tongue in their production while the last four involve the back of the tongue.

Anterior/Nonanterior Anterior/nonanterior are other names for the front and back features of the oral cavity. All front sounds are called anterior and all back sounds are called nonanterior. The demarcation line in English, for example, is between alveolars and palatals. Thus, considering the oral cavity lengthwise with lips as the front end and the velum as the back end, all consonants produced with constriction between the alveolar ridge and the lips are called anterior and all consonants produced with the constriction between the palate and the velum are called nonanterior. English consonants have the following distribution on this feature: all labials /p, b, f, v, m/, all linguadentals /θ, ð/, and all alveolars /t, d, s, z, n, l/ are +anterior. All palatals /r, tʃ, dʒ, ʃ, ʒ, j/ and all velars /k, g, ŋ, h/ are nonanterior. Because vowels do not involve constriction anywhere in the oral cavity, they are all labeled as nonanterior.

Tongue Body Features The three features high, low, and back relate to the position of the body of the tongue. All these projections of the tongue are measured from its neutral position. The neutral position of the tongue has been defined as in the status of producing the vowel [ʌ] in English /bʌt/.

High/nonhigh: High sounds are produced by raising the tongue body higher than its neutral position. The English consonants /tʃ, dʒ, ʃ, w, ʒ, k, g, ŋ/ are considered high and all other consonants as nonhigh.

Low/nonlow: Low sounds are produced by positioning the tongue body lower than the neutral position; nonlow sounds are produced without such a lowering. The English consonant /h/ is considered low. All other consonants are nonlow.

Back/nonback:Back sounds are produced by moving the body of the tongue further back than the neutral position, whereas the nonback sounds are produced without moving the tongue body back from the neutral position. The back consonants of English are /k, g, w, ŋ/. All other consonants are nonback.

Round Rounded sounds are produced with the rounding of lips to form oval or round variable shapes depending on the amount of rounding needed for the production of a given phoneme. In the production of English /ʃ/ and /ʒ/, some degree of lip rounding is considered necessary, although these consonants are palatal. Rounding, according to Chomsky and Halle, may be manifested in any class of sounds. Rounding is not a distinctive feature used for English consonants.

Distributed/Nondistributed Distributed/nondistributed is a place of articulation feature not utilized in characterizing the sounds of the English language. The anterior/nonanterior and coronal/noncoronal classifications account for all the place of articulation distinctions in English. Below is a chart to show how English alveolars, labials, palatals, and velars are distinguished by the hierarchy of the features anterior/nonanterior and coronal/noncoronal. After this chart is presented another chart showing the distributed/nondistributed features.

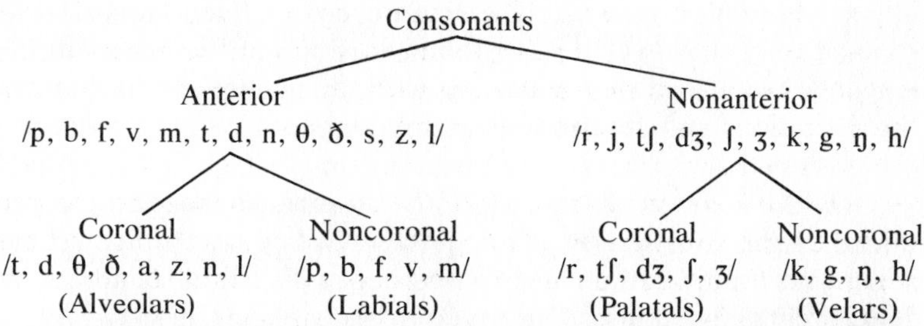

However, assume a language in which the phonological system requires the identification of additional places of articulation. For example, in a language where there are five categories of stops, namely, labial, dental, alveolar, retroflex, and velar, represented, for example, as /p/, /t̪/, /t/, /ṭ/, and /k/, respectively, an additional feature would be needed to distinguish the additional category of the place of articulation feature. Chomsky and Halle described the feature "distributed" to account for such cases. According to Chomsky and Halle (1968, pp. 312–313): "Distributed sounds are produced with a constriction that extends for a considerable distance along the direction of the air flow; nondistributed sounds are produced with constriction that extends only for a short distance in this direction." The distribution of the above stops then would be the following:

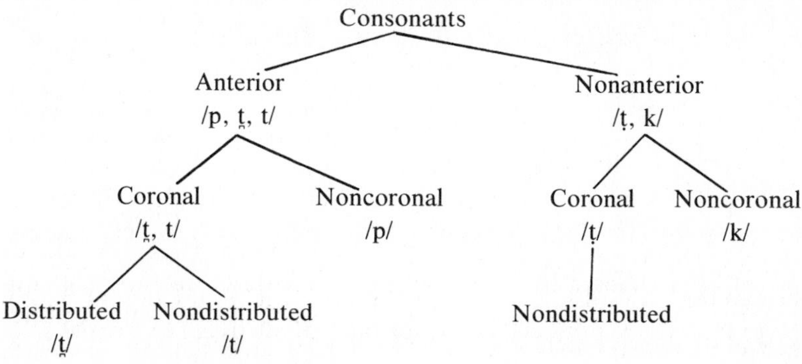

where /t̪/ is distributed and /t/ and /ṭ/ are nondistributed because the production of /t̪/ involves a more extended constriction along the direction of the air flow than the nondistributed consonants /t/ and /ṭ/. Examples of languages that utilize these categories of stop are Hindi and Marathi.

Covered/Noncovered The feature covered/noncovered is restricted only to vowels and is found in some of the West African languages. Because we are dealing with the features of consonants, the definitions and descriptions of covered/noncovered are not presented here.

Glottal Constrictions Glottally constricted sounds are produced by the constriction of the gottal area beyond the neutral narrowing position. Glottal constriction is not a distinctive feature in the English language, but it is in several African languages.

Secondary Apertures There are two categories of secondary apertures: nasal/non-nasal and lateral/nonlateral.

Nasal/non-nasal: Nasals are produced with the lowered velum whereas non-nasals are produced with the velum raised. In English /m, n, ŋ/ are nasal consonants and all other consonants are non-nasal (oral).

Lateral/nonlateral: Lateral consonants are produced by lowering the midsection of the tongue. English possesses vocalic laterals, which are liquid sounds. Nonvocalic laterals are uncommon in the English language. According to Chomsky and Halle (1968, p. 317): "of the laterals only the vocalic (l) occurs with any frequency among the languages of the world." Nonvocalic laterals frequently appear in children with articulation problems of the lateral lisp nature.

Manner of Articulation Features

Continuant/Noncontinuant (Stop) The continuant consonants are produced with the constriction in the vocal tract regulated in such a way that complete closure or blocking of the air passage never occurs. The noncontinuant or the stop consonants, on the other hand, are produced with complete closure or constriction of the vocal tract so that the passage of air is blocked effectively. In English, for the stop plosives, this blocking occurs at three different distinct points: at the lips (for the production of /p, b/), at the alveolar ridge (for the production of /t, d/), and at the velum (for the production of /k, g/). Note that /m, n, ŋ, tʃ, dʒ/ are stops but not plosives. In English, the continuant consonants, according to Chomsky and Halle, are /r, l, f, v, θ, ð, s, z, ʃ, ʒ, h/, and the noncontinuant or stop consonants are /p, b, m, t, d, n, tʃ, dʒ, k, g, ŋ/.

Release Features Two kinds of release features are described by Chomsky and Halle, and both apply to stop consonants only. All stops have a certain amount of release time involved in their production. When the closure in the vocal tract is released, the complete production of the stop consonant is executed. While the plosive stops of English /p, b, t, d, k, g/ are considered as released instantaneously, the affricate stops /tʃ, dʒ/ are considered released with some delay.

Tense/Nontense Among the supplementary features described by Chomsky and Halle, tense/nontense is one used in the English language. While it is necessary to maintain this feature for the vowels of English, for the consonants it is identical to the voicing feature. The consonants that are voiceless /p, t, k, f, θ, s, ʃ, tʃ, h/ are tense and those that are voiced are nontense or lax.

Source Features

Voiced/Voiceless Although Chomsky and Halle discuss thoroughly some acoustic data to investigate the articulatory correlates of the feature voicing, it is safe to assume that their treatment of the feature voicing is similar to ones described earlier: In the production of the voiced consonants, the vocal folds vibrate, and in the production of the voiceless consonants they do not vibrate.

Strident/Nonstrident The definition of strident/nonstrident, according to Chomsky and Halle, is more of an acoustic rather than articulatory nature. They write that strident sounds are marked acoustically by greater noisiness than their nonstrident counterparts. In English, /f, v, s, z, tʃ, dʒ, ʃ, ʒ/ are strident consonants and the rest are nonstridents.

Application of Chomsky and Halle System The Chomsky and Halle feature system applicable only to the English consonants is presented in Table 2-7. Although Chomsky and Halle included 13 features to describe English phonemes, this table includes only 11 features. The features tenseness and voicing are identical for the consonants and therefore only one (voicing) has been included (Chomsky and Halle, 1968, p. 177). The feature rounding specifies the rounding of the sounds /k, g, x/. This phenomenon is eliminated because it is not conventional to use the rounding marker (raised /w/) in the English language to distinguish /k/ from /k^w/ and /g/ from /g^w/, or to use the glottal fricative /x/ and its rounded counterpart /x^w/.

Table 2-7. Chomsky and Halle feature system

Feature	Consonant specification[a]																					
	p	b	t	d	tʃ	dʒ	k	g	f	v	θ	ð	s	z	ʃ	w[b]	r	l	j[b]	h	m	n
Vocalic	0	0	0	0	0	0	0	0	0	0	0	0	0	0	0	0	1	1	0	0	0	0
Consonantal	1	1	1	1	1	1	1	1	1	1	1	1	1	1	1	0	1	1	0	0	1	1
High	0	0	0	0	1	1	1	1	0	0	0	0	0	0	1	1	0	0	1	0	0	0
Back	0	0	0	0	0	0	1	1	0	0	0	0	0	0	0	1	0	0	0	0	0	0
Low	0	0	0	0	0	0	0	0	0	0	0	0	0	0	0	0	0	0	0	1	0	0
Anterior	1	1	1	1	0	0	0	0	1	1	1	1	1	1	0	0	0	1	0	0	1	1
Coronal	0	0	1	1	1	1	0	0	0	0	1	1	1	1	1	0	1	1	0	0	0	1
Voice	0	1	0	1	0	1	0	1	0	1	0	1	0	1	0	1	1	1	1	0	1	1
Continuant	0	0	0	0	0	0	0	0	1	1	1	1	1	1	1	(1)	1	1	(1)	1	0	0
Nasal	0	0	0	0	0	0	0	0	0	0	0	0	0	0	0	(0)	0	0	(0)	0	1	1
Strident	0	0	0	0	1	1	0	0	1	1	0	0	1	1	1	(0)	0	0	(0)	0	0	0

[a] /ʒ/ and /ŋ/ not included in this table. The feature specifications for these two phonemes can be easily extrapolated.
[b] Parenthesized values added.

The categorization implicit in this system can be interpreted at two levels. As binary features, the system specifies the phonemes as they are used in lexical entries. The entries can be quite abstract because complex phonological rules are required to convert them into phonetic representations. These features "provide a representation of an utterance which can be interpreted as a set of instructions to the physical articulatory system, or as a refined level of perceptual representation" (Chomsky and Halle, 1968, p. 65).

A simplified representation of the binary feature system presented in Table 2-7 to interpret the lexical item in a sentence is shown below in Figure 2-2. The attempt in this representation is not to show how these features were extracted by complex phonological rules but to show how these features might be utilized in the coding of lexical items of a sentence. All 13 features of the Chomsky and Halle system for both vowels and consonants are used here because the sentence, *The boy hit the ball,* includes consonants and vowels.

How is a sentence converted into phonological segments? The most simple guess is that syntactic and semantic components generate abstract markers, such as a noun phrase (NP) and a verb phrase (VP), ending with abstract "word" entities called *formatives.* In Figure 2-2, a sentence is generated producing the formatives, *The boy hit the ball.* These five formatives have no perceptual reality to the listener until they are converted into phonetic units. Or, stated in another way, formatives must be converted into physiological segments (phoneme-size units or smaller) in order for speech to result. Exactly how formatives are converted into physiological movements necessary to produce phonetic units is indeed a mystery. However, progress is being made in our understanding of this process.

Distinctive features are regarded as instructions to the speech mechanism. The input to distinctive features is the output of the syntactic generator. The generation of a sentence might proceed as in the following example:

1) S → NP + VP The idea or sentence is rewritten as a noun phrase and a verb phrase.
2) NP → D + N The noun phrase is rewritten as a determiner and a noun.
3) VP → V + NP The verb phrase is rewritten as a verb and a noun phrase.
4) NP → D + N The noun phrase within the predicate is rewritten as a determiner and a noun.

5) D	→	the	A determiner is selected from the lexicon.
6) V	→	hit	A verb is selected from the lexicon.
7) N	→	boy, ball	Nouns are selected from the lexicon.

The syntactic and semantic components generate formatives that are converted into serial sets of distinctive features. At this point we will not comment on the timing relationships involved; that is, we do not know the length of the string over which this process occurs. Obviously, entire sentences are not generated before the initiation of phonetic production. Semantic, syntactic, and phonological constructions, as psychological processes, go on simultaneously, but we know very little about how this takes place.

As mentioned above, the input to phonological segments is the output of the syntactic generator. A word such as *the,* the first word in the sentence depicted in Figure 2-2, would be converted into a column of features as follows: −vocalic, +consonantal, −high, −back, −low, +anterior, +coronal, +voice, +continuant, −nasal, and −strident. If one of the 11 segments in the production of /ð/ were realized incorrectly, a different phoneme would result. For example, if +continuant is produced as −continuant, this phonological set would be uttered as /d/. Within this framework, lexical items such as *the* and *boy* are stored in the memory as an ordered set of phonological features. According to this viewpoint, our mental dictionary stores the word *boy* as a set of columns having the order and composition given in Figure 2-2. Furthermore, because the lexical item *boy* is the input for the three-columnar feature set, the need to store the phonemes /bɔɪ/ seems unnecessary. It can be argued, then, that the basic underlying storage units for lexical items are distinctive features and not phonemes (Chomsky and Halle, 1968).

TRUE PERCEPTUAL FEATURE SYSTEM

Problems with Feature Systems

Some recent advances in a statistical analysis technique have made it possible to search for the "unknown" in the matrices of confusions such as the ones Miller and Nicely, and Singh and Black collected. The problem with the Miller and Nicely, Singh and Black, and Wic-

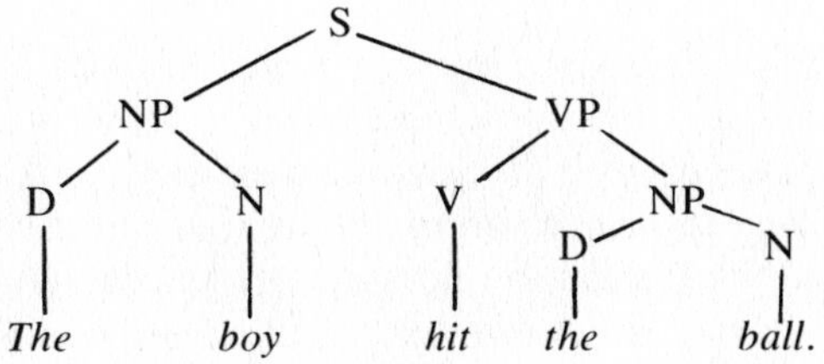

S

NP VP

D N V NP

D N

The *boy* *hit* *the* *ball.*

OR

	ð	ə	b	ɔ	ɪ	h	ɪ	t	ð	ə	b	ɔ	l
Vocalic	−	+	−	+	+	−	+	−	−	+	−	+	+
Consonantal	+	−	+	−	−	−	−	+	+	−	+	−	+
High	−	−	−	−	+	−	+	−	−	−	−	−	−
Back	−	−	−	+	+	−	+	−	−	−	−	+	−
Low	−	−	−	+	−	+	−	−	−	−	−	+	−
Anterior	+	−	+	−	−	−	−	+	+	−	+	−	+
Coronal	+	−	−	−	−	−	−	+	+	−	−	−	+
Round		−		+	+		+			−		+	
Tense		−		+	−		−			−		+	
Voice	+		+			−		−	+		+		+
Continuant	+		−			+		−	+		−		+
Nasal	−		−			−		−	−		−		−
Strident	−		−			−		−	−		−		−

Figure 2-2. A syntactic corpus coded by a distinctive feature system. *S*, sentence; *NP*, noun phrase; *VP*, verb phrase; *D*, determiner; *N* noun; and *V*, verb.

kelgren feature systems is one of arbitrariness. They proposed the feature systems with three considerations:

1. *The features in a system must have articulatory or acoustic references.* For example, in the Miller and Nicely feature system, voicing, nasality, and place of articulation have clear articulation references; the feature affrication can be argued to have articulatory or acoustic references; and the feature duration mainly has acoustic reference.
2. *The features in a system should be sufficient in number and specification to distinguish all consonants of a set with which researchers are working.* Thus, Miller and Nicely had to have five different features (voicing, nasality, affrication, duration, and place of articulation) where four of these had *one* and *zero* (binary) specifications and one (place of articulation) had *three* specifications (*zero, one,* and *two*).
3. *The features of a system should be realistic in the sense that they can be utilized to predict, with the maximal degree of probability, the responses of the subjects' perception of the consonants.* One way to arrive at such a feature system was to inspect the matrices of errors that the consonants generated and then to look for the classes of errors under which the greatest number of confusions occurred. For example, if the voiceless consonants as stimuli yielded voiceless consonants as responses a greater number of times than voiced consonants as responses, voicing was considered a classification of the consonants.

The problem with the above procedure is that it is not possible for an experimenter to eyeball the matrices of a large number of entries (e.g., a confusion matrix consisting of 16 consonants would have 256 entries, where each entry would potentially have different relationships with all the other entries). Additionally, if the consonants would have been investigated in more than one experimental condition (e.g., Miller and Nicely had 17 matrices yielding from 17 experimental conditions, and Singh and Black had 16 matrices yielding from 16 speaking-listening conditions), then the number of different matrices as well as the entries in each matrix would be an impossible task to eyeball and find the classification of the consonants. Therefore, a great deal of arbitrariness existed in the prescriptions of the Miller and Nicely, Singh and Black, and Wickelgren feature systems.

The problem with phonologically derived feature systems, such as that of Chomsky and Halle, and acoustically derived feature systems, such as that of Jakobson, Fant, and Halle, is their postulation that the proposed acoustic and phonological distributions of phonemes are realized in speech production and speech perception. Actually, while a phonologically derived feature system may be satisfactory from a theoretical point of view, if it is unable to account for speech production and speech perception errors, it is not practical to apply such a feature system to the understanding and treatment of phonological problems of deviant speakers. It can be seen later that of the 11 consonant features of the Chomsky-Halle system, one-third had no perceptual relevance. In other words, one-third of the 11 phonological features of Chomsky and Halle were unable to account for any variances in the perceptual errors of the English consonants.

Multidimensional Analysis

In search of a ''true'' feature system that underlies the phonemes of a language, it is necessary to have available as a hypothesis a number of feature systems, e.g., articulatory phonetic features, phonological features, and acoustic features. A statistical technique may be utilized to determine what features are truly realized in the production and the perception of speech sounds. A series of statistical techniques recently used is called the multidimensional scaling procedure. There are several different multidimensional scaling methods. The ones that have been predominately utilized in the speech research are MDSCAL and INDSCAL, both developed at the Bell Telephone Laboratories (Murray Hill, N.J.).

An experimenter sets out to collect similarity or dissimilarity judgments involving a given set of phonemes. The similarity or dissimilarity matrix is generated by one of several methods of eliciting responses. Methods of: 1) absolute judgment (as in Miller and Nicely, and Singh and Black), 2) paired comparison (as in Singh, Woods, and Becker, 1972), and 3) triadic comparison (as in Singh, Woods, and Becker, 1972; and Mitchell and Singh, 1974) have been utilized to determine the proximity of the consonants. In the case of the absolute judgment method, listeners are asked to report what they heard. The greater the number of error responses, the more similar the two consonants are considered. Such a confusion matrix is called a *similarity matrix*. In paired comparison experiments, different psychological methods can be adopted to elicit judgments of the similarity of consonants. Pairs of consonants are presented auditorily, and the subjects are asked to rate them on a given scale, say on a seven-point scale, to determine how similar the sounds of a pair are. The instruction given to the subject is to assign a smaller number on the scale to pairs that are more similar auditorily (the more similar the pair the smaller the number assigned). Thus, if the listener judges no difference between two syllables of a pair, he assigns the value of *one*. If he considers the two pairs farthest apart in his judgment, he assigns the value of *seven*. These values are then used to construct a matrix of the stimulus-response phoneme. For example, if the rating experiment included only six consonants, /p, t, k, b, d, g/, the matrix will have 36 values. Six of these values will involve the identity comparison, for example, the comparisons of /p/ to /p/, /t/ to /t/, etc. Fifteen of the 36 values would involve the comparison of all the six sounds in one order, for example, /p-t/, /p-k/, etc. The other fifteen values will involve the comparison of the same six sounds in the altered order, for example, /t-p/, /k-p/, etc.

A comparison of consonants or vowels by methods of psychological judgments such as the ones above provides a score of relative similarity of the sounds. The more similar the two sounds are, the smaller the value in the matrix. The more dissimilar the two sounds are, the larger the value in the matrix. These values representing the judgments of the listeners are called *proximity* because they are mere approximations of the magnitude of similarity between pairs of sounds of speech. There are several psychological methods that can be utilized to approximate the similarity of phonemes in diads and triads. The essence of all these matrices is to utilize them to discover the perceptual strategies that listeners use when they make proximity judgments. In other words, when the listeners judged /p-t/ as being a more similar pair than /p-g/, what were the bases of their decision?

The multidimensional analysis techniques have been used to find the strategies of the listener-judges in terms of the following critical points:

1. In what dimensional space or in how many dimensions are the consonant (or vowel) phonemes perceived?
2. Are these dimensions, in nature and property, similar to acoustic and/or articulatory features?
3. Do these dimensions contribute equally to the perception, or does some dimension contribute more to the perception of the consonants than another dimension?
4. Do all judges use each dimension, or do some judges use one set of dimensions while other judges use another set of dimensions?
5. Are there differences in the individual ranking of the features of the different judges?

If these questions are answered with reliability, the distinctive feature system obtained from the multidimensional scaling analysis would be the most realistic feature system presently possible for interpreting phonemic responses. Such a feature system has been proposed by Singh, Woods, and Becker (1972) for the 22 consonants of English and further substantiated by Mitchell and Singh (1974), Weiner and Singh (1974), and Danhauer and Singh (1975).

Two different tasks were undertaken by Singh, Woods, and Becker (1972): 1) to test statistically the relative predictive power of some of the existing feature systems, and 2) to obtain a feature system that is "truly" a function of the perceptual responses of the listeners. The feature systems tested were those of Miller and Nicely, Singh and Black, Wickelgren, and Chomsky and Halle. Of the four feature systems tested, the Chomsky and Halle system seemed to correlate most highly. However, when a new feature system was obtained (by the multidimensional scaling procedure) from the actual perceptual responses of the listeners, then that feature system showed higher correlations than the Chomsky and Halle feature system.

Before reporting the feature system obtained from the perceptual data by the statistical technique called multidimensional scaling, other questions raised earlier may be answered in brief. The 22 prevocalic consonants were perceived in three-, four-, or five-dimensional spaces. Each of these dimensions, when plotted geometrically, was interpreted by one phonetic and/or acoustic feature. Thus, in Singh, Woods, and Becker, a five-dimensional solution was interpreted as: dimension 1 = place of articulation (front/back), dimension 2 = sibilancy, dimension 3 = voicing, dimension 4 = plosiveness, and dimension 5 = nasality. The contributions of these five dimensions to the perception of the consonants were different. In other words, these five features maintain different degrees of weights. The rank order from the most important (or strong) dimension to the least important (or weak) dimension is: 1) place of articulation (front/back), 2) nasality, 3) sibilancy, 4) voicing, and 5) plosiveness. It may be added here that the rank order of the features presented is an average of all subjects. In Chapter 5 it will be demonstrated that all subjects do not conform to the above rank orders. As a matter of fact, although all subjects seem to utilize all five features, some subjects may utilize them in one rank order while other subjects utilize them in another rank order.

Based on the interpretations of a five-dimensional multidimensional analysis solution and the phonetic interpretations of each of these dimensions, a five-feature system was obtained by Singh, Woods, and Becker. The following is the description of that feature system.

INDSCAL Feature System Proposed by Singh, Woods, and Becker

Voicing and nasality were identical to the earlier feature systems. The place of articulation feature was identical to the Chomsky and Halle feature anterior (with opposite specifications). The feature sibilancy included /s, z, ʃ, tʃ, dʒ/ as +sibilant and all other consonants as −sibilant. The feature plosiveness classified the six plosives of English /p, t, k, b, d, g/ in one group and the remaining consonants in another. It may be noted that the consonants in the Singh, Woods, and Becker study were presented initially; and at the initial position, English /p, t, k, b, d, g/ are exploded more than at the medial and final positions.

The feature system presented in Table 2-8 is an outcome of three data collection methods involving three groups of adult listeners and the application of multidimensional analysis techniques. The binary specification of all five features is suggested in the distribution of the 22 consonants on the coordinates of the five-dimensional solution. The assignment of 0 and 1 to the two different clusters on a dimension was arbitrary.

There remains a problem with the Singh, Woods, and Becker feature system, a problem that is an artifact of a considerable reliance on the statistical technique to tease out the features of the perceptual or the productive data involving the consonants: The feature system does not contain enough features, and/or sufficient number of specifications of the features, to accommodate the phonological differences of the 22 consonants analyzed. For example, with the existing feature system, the phoneme groups /p-t/, /b-d/, /tʃ-ʃ/, /f-θ/, /v-ð-l/, /w-r-j/, and /m-n/ are indistinctive. As can be recalled, the binary specification of the feature place of articulation is the reason for most of these unities. For example, if labial place were introduced, /p/ would be different from /t/, /b/ from /d/, /f/ from /θ/, /v/ from /ð, l/, /w/ from /r, j/, and /m/ from /n/. The feature stop rather than plosive would enable the distinction of /tʃ/ from /ʃ/. But, unfortunately, there is no good support in the multidimensional scaling analyses of any of the data sets so far (Mitchell and Singh, 1974; Danhauer and Singh, 1975a) to suggest a further breakdown of the front specification of the front/back feature to labial/nonlabial. The Mitchell and Singh study showed the

Table 2-8. INDSCAL (a multidimensional analysis technique) feature system proposed by Singh, Woods, and Becker

Feature	Consonant specification																					
	p	b	t	d	tʃ	dʒ	k	g	f	v	θ	ð	s	z	ʃ	w	r	l	j	h	m	n
Place	0	0	0	0	1	1	1	1	0	0	0	0	0	0	1	1	1	0	1	1	0	0
Nasality	0	0	0	0	0	0	0	0	0	0	0	0	0	0	0	0	0	0	0	0	1	1
Sibilancy	0	0	0	0	1	1	0	0	0	0	0	0	1	1	1	0	0	0	0	0	0	0
Voicing	0	1	0	1	0	1	0	1	0	1	0	1	0	1	0	1	1	1	1	0	1	1
Plosive	1	1	1	1	0	0	1	1	0	0	0	0	0	0	0	0	0	0	0	0	0	0

existence of the velar place feature, which would divide the back consonants into the groups velar and nonvelar.

It may be noted that the multidimensional analysis technique is a very promising tool to retrieve a "true" feature system from the phonemic responses of the speakers and listeners. Whatever features have been found so far also indicate that the perceptual and productive strategies utilize common phonological commands. The features that are common to both speech perception and speech production can be utilized without many restrictions to tackle the problems of both speech production and speech perception. It is evident that some interpretations of the perceptual responses were articulatory in nature. This suggests in the human response system a parsimony of phoneme production and phoneme perception. If this theory is substantiated, then a test of articulation also would serve as a test for speech discrimination, and with this parsimonious approach the bifurcated fields of speech and hearing may start working in a more conjunctive way. After all, if the theory proves that the command to the speech and hearing mechanisms for phoneme production and phoneme perception is given in terms of the distinctive features, then those distinctive features should be the criteria for testing, diagnosing, and constructing therapeutic strategies, and measuring prognosis of both phoneme production and phoneme perception.

chapter 3 Distinctive Feature Systems of Vowels

CONTENTS

Jakobson, Fant, and Halle (1951)
Peterson and Barney (1952)
Phonological feature system of Chomsky and Halle (1968)
Perceptual feature system

There has been less controversy regarding the features of vowels than the features of consonants. Most proponents of the vowel feature system agree about some of the basic properties of the vowel features. Different investigators of the vowel features (Bricker, 1967; Hanson, 1967; Pols, Van der Kamp, and Polmp, 1969; Anglin, 1971; Singh and Woods, 1971; Terbeek and Harshman, 1971; Shepard, 1972) seem to agree on the perceptual features of vowels and the correspondence of the perceptual features with acoustic and articulatory characteristics.

Traditionally, the vowels are described in three-dimensional space where two of the dimensions relate to the horizontal and vertical axes of the human vocal tract and the third dimension is described by a different name depending on the convention that a phonetician may follow. The horizontal dimension of the vowels of English is described as front/central/back and on the vertical dimension they are described as high/mid/low. Figure 3-1 shows an articulatory based diagram of the English vowels. Utilizing this diagram, we can distinguish the vowels /i, ɪ/ as high-front, /e, ɛ/ as mid-front, /æ/ as low-front, /u, ʊ/ as high-back, /o, ɔ/ as mid-back, /ɑ/ as low-back, and /ə, ʌ/ as mid-central. However, in this diagram, no parameter has been described that will distinguish between /i/ and /ɪ/, /e/ and /ɛ/, /u/ and /ʊ/, /o/ and /ɔ/, and /ə/ and /ʌ/. There is evidence in the literature to

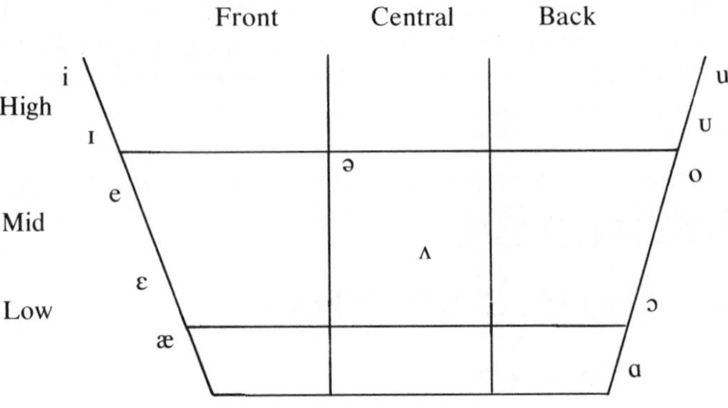

Figure 3-1. An articulatory description of the main English vowels.

support the contention that vowel production is on a continuum. Thus, a more elaborate determination of points on the continuum of height would be to extend the ternary specifications to a quaternary specification. In the pairs of vowels where indistinctions have been shown, it is evident that /i/ consistently is higher than /ɪ/, /e/ higher than /ɛ/, /u/ higher than /ʊ/, /o/ higher than /ɔ/, and /ə/ higher than /ʌ/.

Figure 3-2 shows an alternative articulatory description of the main English vowels. In this description the advancement dimension, while still maintaining the ternary specifications of the front/central/back and height dimensions, now has been characterized by a five-way specification. Thus, instead of high/mid/low, now there

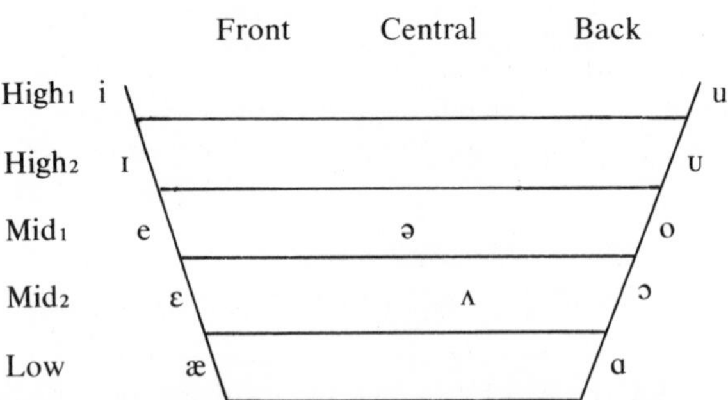

Figure 3-2. An alternative articulatory description of the main English vowels.

are $high_1$/$high_2$/mid_1/mid_2/ and low. It may be pointed out that an alternative description of the height dimension is the continuum of the vocal tract opening, where the high vowels require minimal opening of the tract, with increased opening required as one proceeds from high to low, and with maximal opening for /æ/.

A feature system now can be proposed utilizing the dimensions of advancement (horizontal) and height (vertical) of the human vocal tract. The 12 main vowels can be distinguished each from the other by the ternary advancement and five-way height features. Table 3-1 presents such a feature system.

Table 3-1. Articulation-based distinctive feature system for English vowels

	Vowel specification											
Feature	i	ɪ	e	ɛ	æ	ɑ	ɔ	o	ʊ	u	ə	ʌ
Advancement	1	1	1	1	1	3	3	3	3	3	2	2
Height	5	4	3	2	1	1	2	3	4	5	3	2

Some acoustic phoneticians and phonologists prefer to solve the indistinctions of the pairs /i, ɪ/, /e, ɛ/, /u, ʊ/, /o, ɔ/, and /ə, ʌ/ by the feature *tense/lax,* where the first member of each of these pairs is considered tense and the second member lax. The tense vowels may be described as the ones with higher tongue elevation than their lax counterparts on the height dimension. On the advancement dimension, the tense vowel is slightly more fronted within the advanced (front) category and slightly more retracted within the back vowel category. Tense vowels are generally longer in duration and amplitude than their lax counterparts. Linguistically, tense and lax vowels serve as different bases for formulating the phonological rules of the English vowel system.

A three-feature description of these vowels emerges. The resulting feature system is shown in Table 3-2.

JAKOBSON, FANT, AND HALLE (1951)

Jakobson, Fant, and Halle (1951) described the six English vowels (Received Pronunciation) mainly by the features compact/diffuse,

Table 3-2. Distinctive feature system for English vowels utilizing the features advancement, height, and tenseness

	Vowel specification											
Feature	i	ɪ	e	ɛ	æ	ɑ	ɔ	o	ʊ	u	ə	ʌ
Advancement	1	1	1	1	1	3	3	3	3	3	2	2
Height	3	3	2	2	1	1	2	2	3	3	2	2
Tenseness	1	0	1	0			0	1	0	1	1	0

grave/acute, and flat/plain. Table 3-3 shows the allocation of these features to the six English vowels. According to Jakobson, Fant, and Halle, these six vowels in English can have two manifestations depending on the prosodic opposition stressed vs. unstressed.

The terms *compact/diffuse* and *grave/acute* already have been defined in Chapter 2, in the description of the 21 consonants of English by the Jakobson, Fant, and Halle feature system. The flat vowels manifest a downward trend of the formants of the vowels while the plain vowels do not manifest such a shift.

Table 3-3. Six English vowels described by Jakobson, Fant, and Halle

	Vowel specification					
Feature	o	ɑ	e	u	ə	i
Compact/diffuse	+	+	+	−	−	−
Grave/acute	+	+	−	+	+	−
Flat/plain	+	−		+	−	

PETERSON AND BARNEY (1952)

The acoustic analysis of 10 English vowels was carried out extensively by Peterson and Barney (1952), who had a large group of speakers saying the words *heed, hid, head, had, hod, hawed, hood, who'd, hud,* and *heard,* using the vowels /i, ɪ, ɛ, æ, ɑ, ɔ, ʊ, u, ʌ, and ɝ/, respectively. They used male, female, and child speakers. They analyzed a total of 1,520 words spoken by the 76 speakers. The frequencies of the first two formants (F_1 and F_2) of these vowels were plotted. Although some overlap existed between the vowls /ɝ/ and /ɛ/, /ɝ/ and /ʊ/, /ʊ/ and /u/, and /ɑ/ and /ɔ/, in general the central tendencies of the F_1 and F_2 plottings of all speakers seemed to indicate a correspondence to the articulatory features of the advancement and height dimensions. These findings of Peterson and Barney might have been expected because the formants reflect the resonance characteristics of the vocal tract. The measures of F_1 and F_2 provided an excellent approximation of the vocal tract characteristics of the vowel production. Additionally, the very direct correspondence between the articulatory characteristics of tongue advancement and tongue height and their acoustic correlates F_2 and F_1, respectively, suggested strongly that vowel perception may be explained in terms of the features advancement and height. Whether the perceptual cues may be acoustic or articulatory or both, vowel perception theory would have the identical correspondence to both articulatory and acoustic parameters.

Figure 3-3 shows the central points of the F_1 and F_2 of the 10 English vowels studied by Peterson and Barney. It is clear from these acoustic representations of the English vowels that the F_1 and F_2

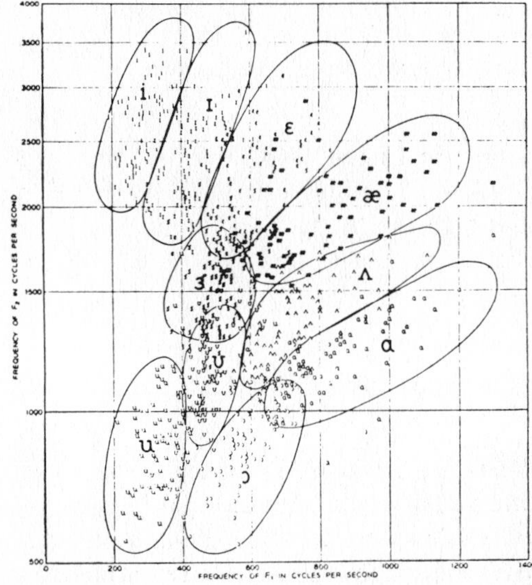

Figure 3-3. Central points of F_1 and F_2 of the 10 English vowels investigated by Peterson and Barney (1952). Frequency of second formant versus frequency of first formant for 10 vowels by 76 speakers. (Reprinted from Peterson and Barney, 1952.)

plottings resemble the articulatory descriptions of the vowels traditionally presented in a vowel diagram.

Table 3-4 shows an acoustic feature system that describes the 12 vowels by the relative height of the F_1 and F_2. In this table, *H* stands for high formant frequencies, *M* stands for mid formant frequencies, and *L* stands for low formant frequencies. If a rank order were used, where the high F frequency would be represented by rank 1, mid F frequency by rank 2, and low F frequency by rank 3, this system then would have a direct correspondence to the articulatory feature system.

Table 3-4. Height of F_1 and F_2 of 12 English vowels as acoustic distinctive parameters

	Height (and rank) of formant frequencies for vowels[a]											
Formant frequencies	i	ɪ	e	ɛ	æ	ɑ	ɔ	o	u	ʊ	ə	ʌ
F_1	L (3)	L (3)	M (2)	M (2)	H (1)	H (1)	M (2)	M (2)	L (3)	L (3)	M (2)	M (2)
F_2	H (1)	H (1)	H (1)	H (1)	H (1)	L (3)	L (3)	L (3)	L (3)	L (3)	M (2)	M (2)

[a]H, high (rank 1); M, mid (rank 2); L, low (rank 3).

Utilizing the specifications in Table 3-4, the vowels /i, ɪ/ would be represented by low F_1 and high F_2; /e, ɛ/ by mid F_1 and high F_2; /æ/ by high F_1 and high F_2; /ɑ/ by high F_1 and low F_2; /ɔ, o/ by mid F_1 and low F_2; /u, ʊ/ by low F_1 and low F_2; and /ə, ʌ/ by mid F_1 and mid F_2.

PHONOLOGICAL FEATURE SYSTEM OF CHOMSKY AND HALLE (1968)

Chomsky and Halle (1968), like Jakobson, Fant, and Halle, described a unitary feature system for both the vowels and consonants. However, the features that were critical in distinguishing vowels had little or no overlap for the consonants. The features high, back, low, round, and tense were used to describe the English vowels.

Table 3-5. Chomsky-Halle vowel feature system

	Vowel specification[a]													
Feature	ī	ū	ē	ō	ǣ	ɑ̄	ɔ̄	i(ɪ)	u(ʊ)	e(ɛ)	ʌ	o	æ	ɔ
High	1	1	0	0	0	0	0	1	1	0	0	0	0	0
Back	0	1	0	1	0	1	1	0	1	0	1	1	0	1
Low	0	0	0	0	1	1	1	0	0	0	0	0	1	1
Round	0	1	0	1	0	0	1	0	1	0	0	1	0	1
Tense	1	1	1	1	1	1	1	0	0	0	0	0	0	0

[a]Bars over the vowels indicate lengthening and diphthongization, e.g., /ī/ as in *why*.

According to Table 3-5, the vowels /ī, ū, i, u/ are high and the remaining vowels are nonhigh; /ū, ō, ɑ̄, ɔ̄, u, ʌ, o, ɔ/ are back and the remaining vowels are nonback; /ǣ, ɑ̄, ɔ̄, æ, ɔ/ are low and the remaining vowels are nonlow; /ū, ō, ɔ̄, u, o, ɔ/ are round and the remaining vowels are nonround; and /ī, ū, ē, ō, ǣ, ɑ̄, ɔ̄/ are tense and the remaining vowels are lax or nontense.

The Chomsky-Halle feature system is binary and hence only two levels of the traditionally three-level height and advancement dimensions are specified. The Chomsky-Halle feature system is unique not so much in positing the features or parameters to describe the vowels as much as in describing the vowels themselves. If viewed from the IPA (International Phonetic Alphabet) point of view, the vowels included in Table 3-5 are /i, u, e, o, æ, ɑ, ɔ, ɪ, ʊ, ɛ, ʌ/. The rest of the vowels, i.e., tense/lax /o/, tense/lax /æ/, and tense/lax /ɔ/, have to be described in terms of their distinct contrastive usage in the English language. Thus, for those who would be interested in using the Chomsky-Halle feature system to code English vowels as a classificatory feature system applied to conventionally designed vowels of English, it is safe to utilize only the 11 vowels whose distinctions are clearly interpretable in a feature vs. IPA vowel matrix. Readers interested in the more advanced treatment of the phonological components of the English vowels should refer to Chomsky and Halle (1968, pp. 178–222).

Chomsky and Halle have used alternate rules to explain different phonetic manifestations of the selected English vowels. Thus, for example, the tense/lax alterations would permit the vowel contrast in in words such as duti/dutɪfəl, mitɚ/mɛtrɪk, minɪŋ/mɛnt, etc., where /i/ in *duty* is tense and /ɪ/ in *dutiful* is lax; /i/ in *meter* is tense and /ɛ/ in *metric* is lax; and /i/ in *meaning* is tense and /ɛ/ in *meant* is lax. Although these alterations are interesting and form the basis of English vowel phonology, a student of speech and hearing pathology may be interested only in the different distinctive feature properties of these vowels and not in uncovering the historical and analytical bases of the English vowel system. Thus, because tense/lax opposition exists in English vowels such as beat/bit, and via the alternate examples that Chomsky and Halle have suggested, the tense/lax feature is utilized to group the 11 vowels of English as /i, u, e, o/ tense, /ɪ, ʊ, ɛ, ʌ/ lax, and /æ, ɑ, ɔ/ either tense or lax depending on their usage in word context and not particularly marked for either.

High/Low

According to the Chomsky-Halle vowel feature system, the vowels /i, u, ɪ, ʊ/ are high and the rest are nonhigh while the vowels /æ, ɑ, ɔ/ are low and the rest are nonlow. The high and low dimensions are functions of the height and lowering of the tongue while producing these vowels. Thus, while in the production of /i, u, ɪ, ʊ/ the tongue is elevated in the vocal tract, in the production of the remaining vowels this elevation is not crucial. Similarly, in the production of the vowels /æ, ɑ, ɔ/ the extreme lowering of the tongue is an important distinctive feature, while in the production of the remaining vowels this lowering does not occur.

Back/Rounded

While the back/nonback dimension of the Chomsky-Halle vowel description is a function of the traditionally described tongue advancement dimension, because of the binary description of their vowels, Chomsky and Halle have pooled the traditionally described central vowels in one of two groups. The vowels /u, o, ɑ, ɔ, ʊ, ʌ/ are considered back and /i, ɪ, e, ɛ, æ/ as nonback. Rounding is a function of the back vowels only. Rounding implies the rounding of the lips while producing the back vowels. Thus, using the Chomsky-Halle system we may describe the 11 vowels in the following tree diagram system:

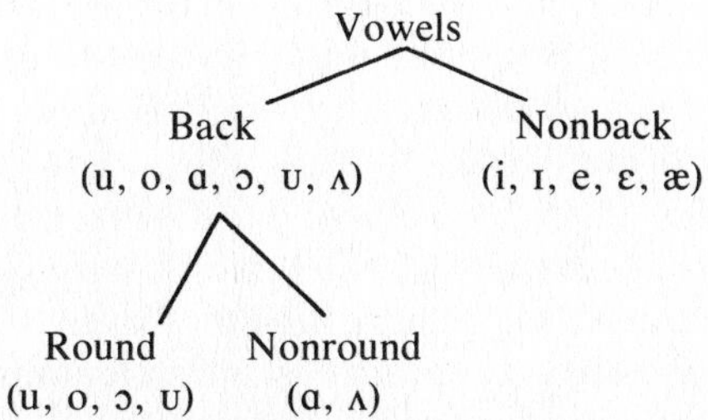

The Chomsky-Halle feature system when interpreted at the segmental level utilizing IPA is essentially similar to the traditional phonetic features. The primary differences lie in the adherence to the binary rather than ternary features of height and advancement. It is mainly because of this principle that Chomsky and Halle had to introduce high/nonhigh and low/nonlow instead of the one feature of height with three specifications. A close examination of these tongue height features reveals that the vowels /i, u, ɪ, ʊ/ are high, the vowels /æ, ɑ, ɔ/ are low, and the vowels /e, ɛ, o, ʌ/ are neither high nor low. Because the dimensions of vowel production are considered a continuum, apparently the vowels that are nonhigh and nonlow are the mid vowels. The traditional articulatory vowel diagram describes the vowels /e, ɛ, ə, ʌ/ as mid. Similar is the case with the feature rounding. The back/rounded feature has been introduced to account for those central vowels that cannot be described by the back/nonback feature. The vowels /ɑ, ʌ/ are somewhere in the central position of the vocal tract rather than located either at the front or the back.

PERCEPTUAL FEATURE SYSTEM

More recently, the vowels of English (and of some other languages) have been investigated perceptually. The hypothesis tested in these recent studies has been that the known acoustic and/or articulatory parameters of the vowels may be utilized as the perceptual cues. One of the earlier studies involved the reanalysis of the Peterson and Barney matrices of the perception of the English vowels.

Shepard (1972) analyzed the perceptual responses (the confusion matrices) of the 10 Peterson and Barney vowels by a multidimensional analysis procedure. The multidimensional analysis procedure is designed to tease out the appropriate perceptual dimension utilized by the subjects in making judgments about the vowels. Shepard reported a two-dimensional solution of the Peterson and Barney vowel matrix. The dimensions were interpreted as the tongue advancement and tongue height features with the three levels of specifications of both of the features. Thus, the 10 vowels clustered into groups of three on the advancement dimension, yielding the feature specifications front/central/back, and also clustered into three groups on the height dimension, yielding high/mid/low.

Shepard's findings alluded to a parsimonious vowel system where the perception of the vowels of English was described by both the formant characteristics and the articulatory descriptions of the vowels. It may be recalled that, while the height feature related to the F_1 frequencies of the vowel, the advancement feature related to the F_2 frequencies. Thus, the reference to vowel perception was present in the articulatory data which have precise acoustic descriptions available in the literature.

This theory of vowel perception is interesting and therefore it is deemed necessary to examine some of the results of vowel perception in languages other than English. Recent work of Hanson (1967), involving Swedish vowels, analyzed the responses of the subjects by a statistical analysis technique (factor analysis) that revealed the relevant dimensions of the vowel perception. Singh and Woods (1971) and Terbeek and Harshman (1971) studied the English vowels perceptually and retrieved their perceptual dimensions via different multidimensional analysis techniques. Anglin (1971) studied the English vowels in the context of words. The results of all these studies are fairly consistent and in keeping with the articulatory, acoustic, and phonological descriptions of the vowel systems.

Singh and Woods (1971) analyzed the subjects' judgments of similarities of the main vowels of English and discovered that the native speakers of English perceived vowels in a three-dimensional space. The first dimension was advancement, where the vowels clustered in three groups, yielding distinctions of front/central/back. The second dimension was height, again yielding three different clusters of high/mid/low. The third dimension was retroflexion, which separated a unitary vowel /ɝ/ from all other vowels. Figure 3-4 shows the output of the multidimensional analysis of the perceptual judgments of the main English vowels. Figure 3-4 shows only 11 English vowels because the vowel /ɝ/ was eliminated for one set of analysis. The interpoint distances, location, and the orientations of these 11 vowels

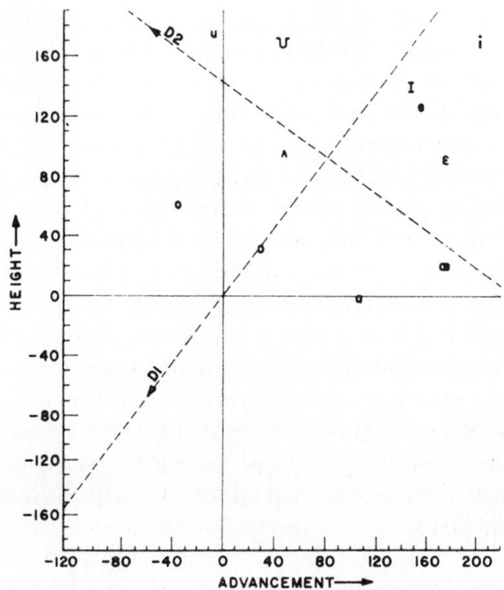

Figure 3-4. Output of multidimensional analysis of perceptual judgments of main English vowels from data by Singh and Woods (1971). Rotation of two-dimensional configuration of MDSCAL output. (Reprinted from Singh and Woods, 1971.)

are precisely a result of how the subjects judged these vowels. If one recalls an articulatory vowel diagram or the associated plottings of the F_1 and F_2 of the vowels, the perceptual configurations mirror those diagrams. Thus, on dimension 1, the vowels /i, ɪ, e, ɛ, æ/ cluster together, the vowels /ɑ, ʌ/ are somewhat in the central area, and the vowels /u, ʊ, o, ɔ/ cluster at the opposite end. Viewing from the top of this figure, /u, ʊ, i, ɪ/ are represented by the highest points (on dimension 2) and the vowels /æ, ɑ, ɔ/ by the lowest points. The remaining vowels are neither high nor low and are labeled as mid.

These results are striking in the sense that they not only explain the contributions of articulatory and acoustic references to vowel perception but also show a concordance with the Chomsky-Halle vowel features that were extracted by examining the lexical entries of the English language. For example, an alternative strategy for interpreting the clusters in Figure 3-4 would be to consider the vowels /i, ɪ, e, ɛ, æ/ (front) as one cluster group and the vowels /u, ʊ, ʌ, o, ɔ, ɑ/ (back) as another cluster group. Within the second cluster groups, the vowels /u, ʊ, o, ɔ/ may be considered rounded and the vowels /ɑ, ʌ/ as unrounded, the vowels /u, ʊ, i, ɪ/ as high and the rest as nonhigh, and the vowels /æ, ɑ, ɔ/ as low and the rest as nonlow. These descriptions are in total agreement with the Chomsky and Halle description of these vowels. It may be noted also that the points that the vowels have assumed in a two-dimensional space are fixed, and the only interpretation that can be superimposed on this diagram would be the one that does not violate the points. Thus, if one were to examine the *y* coordinate the vowels /u, ʊ, ɪ, i/ would have higher values than any other vowels of the set, and the vowels /æ, ɑ, ɔ/ would have lower values than any other vowels of the set. Similarly, if one were to view the *x* axis, the vowels /i, ɪ, e, ɛ, æ/ would have higher values and the vowels /u, ʊ, ʌ, o, ɔ/ would have lower values than any other vowels of the set. In other words, the clusters represented here are the result of the multidimensional analysis.

The above description applies only to the 11 vowels of English. When a 12th vowel, namely, /ɝ/, was added, the analysis resulted in a three-dimensional space, where the vowel /ɝ/ alone belonged to the third dimension.

It may be recalled that the descriptions of the ternary features of advancement and height do not provide a distinction between the vowel pairs /i, ɪ/, /u, ʊ/, and /e, ɛ/. The feature suggested by Chomsky and Halle and others is tenseness. The vowels /i, u, e/ are tense and the vowels /ɪ, ʊ, ɛ/ are lax. When this classification of the vowels was tested against the Singh and Woods (1971) data, a poor correlation resulted. In other words, the feature tenseness was not retrieved perceptually in the Singh and Woods study. For a possible explanation, it was argued that the absence of the emergence of tenseness as a perceptual feature in the Singh and Woods study might have been the function of the isolated sustained vowels as stimuli.

It is not easy to keep the laxness feature intact, for example, and sustain a lax vowel in isolation. This assumption was tested as hypothesis by Anglin (1971). She presented the main English vowels in the context of English words (the context used by Peterson and Barney, namely, /hʌd/). A multidimensional analysis of the subjects' responses of the similarity of these vowels yielded a four-dimensional solution. The first dimension was advancement, the second height, the third retroflexion, and the fourth dimension was tenseness. Thus, when presenting the vowels in the interconsonantal context, Anglin recovered solutions identical to those that Singh and Woods had recovered for the isolated vowels plus an extra dimension interpreted as tenseness. Thus, the conclusion was that the features advance-

Table 3-6. A perceptual feature system of English vowels

	Vowel specification											
Feature	i	ɪ	e	ɛ	æ	ɑ	ɔ	o	ʊ	u	ʌ	ɝ
Advancement	1	1	1	1	1	3	3	3	3	3	2	2
Height	3	3	2	2	1	1	2	2	3	3	2	2
Retroflexion	0	0	0	0	0	0	0	0	0	0	0	1
Tenseness	1	0	1	0	0	1	0	1	0	1	0	1

ment, height, and retroflexion are functions of both isolated and context vowels, but the feature tenseness is a function of context alone.

Table 3-6 shows the vowel feature system that is the result of the combined studies of Singh and Woods, and Anglin. Except for the introduction of the feature retroflexion, the remaining features of this system are consistent with the previously presented and well accepted articulatory and acoustic (F_1-F_2) parameters of the English vowels. This system is perceptual as it is solely a result of subjects' perceptions of the English vowels.

chapter 4
Comparison of Consonant Feature Systems

CONTENTS

Nasality and voicing
Place of articulation
Continuancy
Stridency
Voicing
Duration
Anterior, coronal, grave, and compact
High and back
Liquid, glide, and retroflex
Openness, stop, and continuant

It may be intriguing to readers to discover that the constant set of consonants of the English language has been described by different feature systems in almost completely different manners. The difference among the feature systems lies mainly in the basis of the definition of a phoneme. In other words, the criterion or basis of a phoneme can be acoustic (as in Jakobson, Fant, and Halle), articulatory (as in Chomsky and Halle), or perceptual (as in Singh, Woods, and Becker). Other differences include whether or not the features of the system are strictly binary (as the Jakobson, Fant, and Halle and the Chomsky and Halle systems) or a combination of binary and *n*-ary (ternary, quaternary, etc.) features (as in the Miller and Nicely and the Wickelgren feature systems). It is obvious by now that different feature systems utilize a different number of features. The Wickelgren system utilizes four features, the Miller and Nicely five features, and the Chomsky and Halle 11 features for the consonants of English. Although some features are used consistently in all feature systems (e.g., voicing and nasality), other features have different names and definitions—not very helpful in the overall understanding of the role and reality of the distinctive features in the act of speech production and speech perception.

Table 4-1 lists 23 different features utilized by the proponents of seven different feature systems to describe a maximum of 25 English consonants. There has to be a great deal of overlap among these 23 different features. There are more disagreements rather than agreements among the seven proponents of the seven distinctive feature systems regarding what features should be used to describe the consonant phonemes of English. Twelve features, namely, anterior, coronal, sibilant, tense, liquid, glide, retroflex, openness, high, back, low, and plosive, have been utilized by only one of the seven postulators of these feature systems. Four features, namely, duration, compact, affrication, and grave, have been utilized two out of seven times. The features vocalic, consonantal, continuant, and strident have been used three times each, the feature place four times, voicing six times, and nasality seven times each out of a total possibility of seven.

From Table 4-1 it is clear that the maximal number of features (11) were used by Chomsky and Halle and the minimal number of features (four) were used by Wickelgren. Both Miller and Nicely, and Singh, Woods, and Becker used five features each. Jakobson, Fant, and Halle, Halle, and Singh and Black used eight features each.

NASALITY AND VOICING

The feature nasality was common to all feature systems. The feature voicing was common to six of the seven feature systems. The Jakobson, Fant, and Halle (JFH) feature system treated the feature voicing by the feature tenseness. Thus, in JFH, all English unvoiced consonants were considered +tense and all English voiced consonants were considered −tense.

PLACE OF ARTICULATION

The feature place of articulation was treated differently by the different feature systems. Miller and Nicely considered place as a three-category feature, front, mid, and back. The 16 English consonants that they used were divided as place-0 = /p, b, f, v, m/; place-1 = /t, d, θ, ð, s, z, n/; and place-2 = /ʃ, ʒ, k, g/. Thus, they grouped labials as place-0, alveolars as place-1, and palatals and velars as place-2. Singh and Black reclassified the feature place to a four-category

Table 4-1. Use of features in different feature systems

Feature	Jakobson, Fant, and Halle	Miller and Nicely	Halle	Singh and Black/Singh	Wickelgren	Chomsky and Halle	Singh, Woods, and Becker	Number of times a feature appeared
Nasality	+	+	+	+	+	+	+	7
Voicing		+	+	+	+	+	+	6
Place		+		+	+		+	4
Vocalic	+		+			+		3
Consonantal	+		+			+		3
Continuant	+		+			+		3
Strident	+		+			+		3
Duration		+		+				2
Compact	+		+					2
Affrication		+		+				2
Anterior						+		1
Coronal						+		1
Sibilant							+	1

continued.

Table 4-1. (*continued*)

Feature	Jakobson, Fant, and Halle	Miller and Nicely	Halle	Singh and Black/ Singh	Wickelgren	Chomsky and Halle	Singh, Woods, and Becker	Number of times a feature appeared
Grave	+		+					2
Tense	+							1
Liquid				+				1
Glide				+				1
Retroflex				+				1
Openness					+			1
High						+		1
Back						+		1
Low						+		1
Plosive							+	1
Total number of features used for consonants	8	5	8	8	4	11	5	49

feature where a new category subdivided the palatals from the velars. Then, according to the Singh and Black feature system, the 16 Miller and Nicely consonants would be divided into place-1 = /p, b, f, v, m/; place-2 = /t, d, θ, ð, s, z, n/; place-3 = /ʃ, ʒ/; and place-4 = /k, g/. Wickelgren added another category to the feature place of articulation. According to him, place-1 = /p, b, f, v, m/; place-2 = /t, d, θ, ð, n/; place-3 = /s, z/; place-4 = /ʃ, ʒ/; and place-5 = /k, g/. Singh, Woods, and Becker divided place as a binary feature where /p, b, f, v, m, n, t, d, θ, ð, s, z/ were labeled place-1 and /ʃ, ʒ, k, g/ place-2. This definition was identical to the Chomsky-Halle specifications of the English consonants by the feature anterior. Chomsky and Halle labeled /p, b, f, v, m, n, t, d, θ, ð, s, z/ as +anterior and /ʃ, ʒ, k, g/ as −anterior.

The remaining two feature systems, namely, JFH and Halle, treated place as strictly binary. They devised a two-level definition of the feature place of articulation. They accounted for three places of articulation, namely, front, mid, and back categories, by devising compact/diffuse and grave/acute descriptions. First, the back consonants /ʃ, ʒ, k, g/ are considered compact, and the front consonants /p, b, f, v, m, t, d, n, θ, ð, s, z/ are considered diffuse. Of the diffuse consonants, labials /p, b, f, v, m/ are considered grave, and intradentals and alveolars /t, d, θ, ð, s, z, n/ are considered acute. Thus, these features can be reinterpreted in terms of the place of articulation by collapsing the two levels of treatment. Halle, and Jakobson, Fant, and Halle, treated the place of articulation in three categories: front, mid, and back. Because they were using binary systems, they first separated back from front and then subdivided the front into groups of labials and alveolars.

Table 4-2 shows the treatment of the feature place of articulation by the different proponents of the feature systems. The different allocations of the specifications of place to the consonants are a result of various factors. The systems that were strictly committed to binary specifications of all features had to treat the place of articulation on more than one level by more than one feature. For example, Chomsky and Halle treated place on the levels of anterior/posterior, coronal/noncoronal, and back/nonback. Miller and Nicely grouped the labials (including bilabials and labiodentals) in the same group because, they said, the labial stops /p, b/ and labiodental fricatives /f, v/ are distinguished on the stop/fricative continuum rather than the place of articulation continuum. Miller and Nicely pooled together /t, d/, /θ, ð/, and /s, z/. As can be seen in Table 4-2, although Singh and Black agreed with the above grouping, Wickelgren disagreed and

Table 4-2. Place of articulation feature treated by six different feature systems

Study	Place specification for consonants															
	p	b	t	d	k	g	f	v	θ	ð	s	z	ʃ	ʒ	m	n
Miller and Nicely	0	0	1	1	2	2	0	0	1	1	1	1	2	2	0	1
Singh and Black	1	1	2	2	4	4	1	1	2	2	2	2	3	3	1	2
Wickelgren	1	1	2	2	5	5	1	1	2	2	3	3	4	4	1	2
Singh, Woods, and Becker	1	1	1	1	2	2	1	1	1	1	1	1	2	2	1	1
Chomsky and Halle	1	1	1	1	2	2	1	1	1	1	1	1	2	2	1	1
JFH/Halle[a]	1	1	2	2	3	3	1	1	2	2	2	2	3	3	1	2

[a]In JFH and Halle place is a result of combining compactness and gravity.

labeled /s, z/ as having a different place than /θ, ð, t, d, n/. Singh, Woods, and Becker also consider place as a binary feature. Because their feature system is a statistically derived one, they had no provision for separating the labials from the alveolars, as Miller and Nicely and others have done.

Miller and Nicely, JFH, and Halle consider place as labial, alveolar, and back consonants, which include the palatals and velars. The basis of the JFH and Halle systems was the similar frequency composition of the back consonants. Singh and Black separated the back into the palatals and velars, assigning the third and fourth specifications, respectively. Wickelgren also separated them, assigning them fourth and fifth specifications, respectively. It may be noted here that, although there were some bases for the assignments of different specifications to the place of articulation, by and large they were arbitrary in nature (except Chomsky and Halle, and Singh, Woods, and Becker, where Chomsky and Halle were constrained by phonological derivations of the lexical items and Singh, Woods, and Becker by the statistical technique that provided the feature system). It has been a pressing need, therefore, to test the relevance of the different feature systems against speech production and perception and find out which of the above specifications—e.g., a two-way, three-way, four-way, or five-way specification of the feature place—is actually realized.

The features vocalic and consonantal are unique in the JFH, Halle, and the Chomsky and Halle feature systems. All consonants except /w, h, j/ are nonconsonantal in these systems. It may be noted here that two consonants, /w, j/, were treated as glides in the Singh and Black feature system and by the third degree of openness in the Wickelgren feature system. The JFH, Halle, and Chomsky and Halle systems considered /l, r/ as vocalic and all other consonants as nonvocalic. In the Singh and Black feature system, /r, l/ were treated as retroflex and liquid, respectively, and in the Wickelgren system, they were treated as openness-3.

CONTINUANCY

Continuancy in the JFH, Halle, and Chomsky and Halle feature systems is treated as affrication in Miller and Nicely, frication (except /tʃ, dʒ/) in Singh and Black, openness-2 in Wickelgren, and nonplosive (except /tʃ, dʒ, m, n, j, r, l, w/) in Singh, Woods, and Becker. In other words, the consonants that have been traditionally called fricatives are considered continuants by the JFH, Halle, and Chomsky and Halle feature systems. Wickelgren's definition of openness-2 is contrasted from his openness-1 assignment to stops and openness-3 assignment to sonorants. Implicit in this definition is the fact that stops involve a complete closure in the vocal tract, fricatives involve a slight opening (traditionally /f, v, θ, ð/ are called slit fricatives and /s, z, ʃ, ʒ/ grooved fricatives), and sonorants involve a considerable opening in the vocal tract.

STRIDENCY

The feature stridency includes the consonants /f, v, s, z, ʃ, ʒ, tʃ, dʒ/. This feature was introduced by Jakobson, Fant, and Halle and was incorporated in the Halle and the Chomsky and Halle systems. In terms of its comparison with the traditional classification fricative, the strident category leaves out the three fricatives of English, namely, /θ, ð, h/, and adds the affricatives /tʃ, dʒ/. In terms of the comparison of stridency with the feature continuancy, again, stridency leaves out the plus continuants /θ, ð, h/ and adds the minus continuants /tʃ, dʒ/. The feature has mainly an acoustic base in all feature systems. Chomsky and Halle attempted to provide an articulatory description to the sounds of this class, but their description seems to be a very complex articulatory one. The following is their articulatory description of the category stridency (Chomsky and Halle, 1968, p. 329):

> When the air stream passes over a surface, a certain amount of turbulance will be generated depending upon the nature of the surface, the rate of flow, and the angle of incidence. A rougher surface, a faster rate of flow, and angle of incidence closer to ninety degrees will all contribute to greater stridency.

It may be noted here that the subsequent test of the feature stridency as a feature that has been realized as a true parameter of perception and production has yielded negative results. It has been concluded by Singh, Woods, and Becker (1972) that the feature sibilancy, which includes /s, z, ʃ, ʒ, tʃ, dʒ/, has a significantly greater perceptual relevance than the feature stridency.

VOICING

Voicing is one of the very few features that has been accepted by all feature systems. The only exception is one of nomenclature: The Jakobson, Fant, and Halle feature system utilizes the term *tenseness* to represent the category of voicing. All the voiceless consonants are specified as +tense and all the voiced consonants are specified as −tense. This enabled JFH to use one parameter to describe both vowels and consonants. It can be recalled that in English some vowel pairs, e.g., /i, ɪ/, /u, ʊ/, /ɔ, o/, and /e, ɛ/, are distinguished by the feature tenseness. Chomsky and Halle, however, used the terms "voicing" to describe the consonants and "tenseness" to describe the vowels, thus accepting a more traditional viewpoint that, in the distinction of consonants, it is voicing that is crucially important: the lack of vocal fold vibration vs. the presence of vocal fold vibration. In the distinction of the vowels, however, it is the feature tenseness that distinguishes certain pairs.

DURATION

Miller and Nicely used the feature duration to distinguish /s, ʃ, z, ʒ/ from the other fricatives such as /f, v, θ, ð, h/ and assumed that the former have longer duration than the latter. The feature duration is closest to the feature sibilancy. Sibilancy includes two additional sounds, namely, /tʃ, dʒ/. Duration also can be compared with stridency, which includes four other sounds, namely, /f, v, tʃ, dʒ/.

ANTERIOR, CORONAL, GRAVE, AND COMPACT

Chomsky and Halle proposed the features anterior and coronal and showed that the traditional points of articulation can be supplanted by the features anterior and coronal in the following fashion:

	Labial	*Dental*	*Palato-alveolar*	*Velar*
Anterior	+	+	−	−
Coronal	−	+	+	−

or:

	+Coronal	*−Coronal*
+Anterior	Dental	Labial
−Anterior	Palatoalveolar	Velar

Thus, the traditional points of articulation, e.g., labials /p, b, f, v, m, w/, are +anterior and −coronal, the dentals /θ, ð, t, d, n, s, z, l/ are +anterior and +coronal, the palatoalveolars /ʃ, ʒ, tʃ, dʒ, r, j/ are −anterior and +coronal, and the velars /k, g, ŋ, h/ are −anterior and −coronal.

The features grave and acute as well as the features compact and diffuse also can be described in terms of the features anterior and coronal. The following is the relationship of the features anterior and coronal to the features gravity and compactness:

	Grave	*Acute*	*Compact*	*Diffuse*
Anterior			–	+
Coronal	–	+		

The anterior consonants are −compact and +diffuse, and the coronal consonants are −grave and +acute. Blanks are left when the feature is inappropriate; e.g., there is a blank under "compact" for coronal because coronal cannot be described in terms of compact/diffuse. Although some of the compacts, namely, /ʃ, ʒ, tʃ, dʒ, j/, are +coronal, the other compacts, e.g., /k, g, ŋ/, are −coronal. Similarly, although some of the diffuse consonants, namely, /θ, ð, t, d, s, z, n, l/, are +coronal, the other diffuse consonants, e.g., /p, b, f, v, m/, are −coronal.

Chomsky and Halle (1968, p. 306) presented a comparison of the cavity features that they proposed with that of the earlier proposed features: diffuseness, compactness, and gravity. In the following quotation, Chomsky and Halle present several relevant comparisons and rationales:

> 1) Features specifying the position of the body of the tongue are now the same for vowels and consonants.
>
> 2) In the characterization of vowel articulations, the features "high," "low," "back," correspond to the earlier "diffuse," "compact," and "grave," respectively . . .
>
> 3) The feature "anterior" mirrors precisely the feature "diffuse" in consonants.
>
> 4) The feature "coronal" corresponds most closely to the feature "grave" in consonants but with opposite value. Except for the palatals, the consonants that are classified as nongrave in the earlier framework are coronal in the revised framework, whereas those that were classified as grave are noncoronal. The palatals, which in the earlier framework were nongrave, are noncoronal.

HIGH AND BACK

Palatals and velars were +high in the traditional articulatory descriptions of consonants. In the Jakobson, Fant, and Halle and the Halle frameworks, high is regarded as compact, namely, /ʃ, ʒ, tʃ, dʒ, k, g, ŋ, j/. In the Miller and Nicely feature system, this category was considered place-3. In the Singh and Black feature system /ʃ, ʒ, tʃ, dʒ, j/

were labeled as place-3 and /k, g, ŋ/ as place-4, etc. The feature back describes the articulatory position velar place and includes the consonants /k, g, ŋ/.

LIQUID, GLIDE, AND RETROFLEX

The categories liquid, glide, and retroflex were utilized in the Singh feature system. One drawback of these categories is that they were introduced as a feature to account for a very few consonantal entries. Liquid distinguished between only two consonants, namely, /r, l/; glide distinguished between three, namely, /w, j, ʍ/; and retroflex distinguished only one, namely, /r/. The feature sonorancy—found in the perceptual analysis of the consonants in some recent studies (Singh, Woods, Tishman, 1972; Mitchell and Singh, 1974)—has pooled all these categories into one. Sonorant consonants are voiced; /m, n, ŋ, r, l, w, j/ are sonorant and all other consonants are obstruent.

OPENNESS, STOP, AND CONTINUANT

A complete characterization of the sonorant/obstruent category has been presented by Wickelgren, who has used the three degrees of the openness at the point of contact of the articulators to distinguish the traditional phonetic categories of stops, continuants, and sonorants. Stop has the zero degree of openness, continuants have a relatively small degree of openness, and the sonorants have the maximal openness at the point of constriction in the human vocal tract.

The following diagram shows more clearly the classification of consonants in terms of the relative degree of the aperture at the point of constriction:

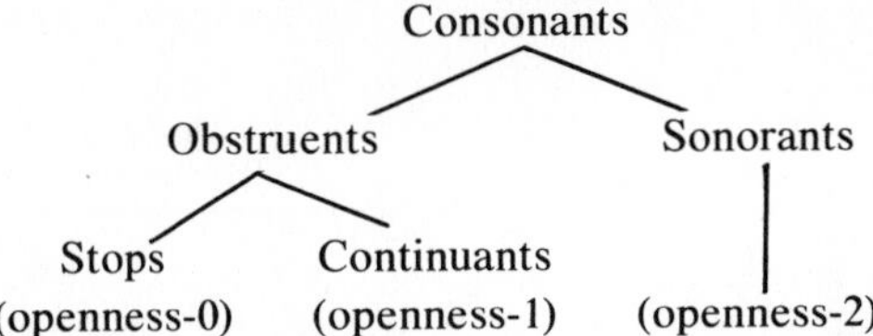

The category of openness takes into consideration the articulatory gesture *aperture* and treats the different traditional manner features on a given continuum, namely, opening. Consistent with the differing degrees of openness of the vowels, this feature continues to increase the number of the specifications of openness. This category treats different consonants and vowels on one continuum.

Role of Distinctive Features in Speech Perception

chapter 5
Distinctive Features in Consonant Perception

CONTENTS

A priori designation of a feature system to predict phoneme perception
Prediction of one set of perceptual responses by one feature system
Prediction of different sets of perceptual responses by a number of feature systems
Role of distinctive features in dichotic processing of the phoneme
A posteriori studies
Retrieval of distinctive features by factor analysis and other spatially less defined methods
Retrieval of distinctive features by INDSCAL
Conclusions
Independence of perceptual features
Satisfaction of certain general criteria for a theory

The phonemes of a language are perceived in terms of distinctive features. The focal point of this chapter is to present categorically a synopsis of those experiments that measure the role of distinctive features in the perception of consonants. The survey of literature pertaining to the role of distinctive features in speech perception strongly supports the reality of the features. The ultimate goal in this chapter is to propose a theory of speech perception based solely on the psychological reality of distinctive features.

Parts of this chapter appeared in S. Singh, ''Distinctive Features: A Measure of Consonant Perception,'' Chapter 3 in *Measurement Procedures in Speech, Hearing, and Language* (edited by S. Singh), University Park Press, Baltimore, 1975.

A PRIORI DESIGNATION OF A FEATURE SYSTEM TO PREDICT PHONEME PERCEPTION

Prediction of One Set of Perceptual Responses by One Feature System

The choice of a given feature system was not adequately explained in a number of studies investigating the perceptual reality of distinctive features. These investigators used one or more competing sets of a priori feature systems to predict listeners' responses to speech sounds. These feature systems are being referred to as a priori because the experimenters determined before the analysis how the data would be classified. The merit of these studies is that they have tested the perceptual importance of a given feature system as a whole and also the relative importance of a feature in a given feature system. These tests have been conducted to determine the rank order of the perceptual strength of the distinctive features in: 1) conditions of acoustic distortion (e.g., noise and filtering) of the stimuli (Miller and Nicely, 1955); 2) cross-linguistic settings (Singh and Black, 1966); 3) the recall of speech sound in short-term memory (Wickelgren, 1966; Klatt, 1968); 4) the utilization of choice reaction time as a measure of distinctive feature differences between phonemes (Cole and Scott, 1972; Weiner and Singh, 1974); and 5) judgment of pairs and triads of speech stimuli utilizing various psychological methods for eliciting perceptual responses (Singh 1970b, 1971; Singh and Becker, 1972; Wang and Bilger, 1973). While all of the above studies prove unambiguously that all features of a given system are not of equal importance, they do not agree regarding the explanatory powers of a given feature system.

Miller and Nicely (1955) Before presenting their experimental results, Miller and Nicely (1955) expressed dissatisfaction with the prevalent method of reporting perceptual responses as a function of noise and frequency distortions. They reported: "One limitation of the existing studies, however, is that results are given almost exclusively in terms of the articulation scores, the percentages of the spoken words that the listener hears correctly. By implication, therefore, all of the listeners' errors are treated as equivalent and no knowledge of the perceptual confusions is available" (p. 388). Thus, instead of eliciting right/wrong or all-or-none types of responses, Miller and Nicely elicited total confusions occurring among the 16 English consonants studied in the context of the vowel /a/ spoken and listened to by five female North American speakers in 17 signal-to-noise (S/N) ratios and filter conditions. Five features with acoustic and articulatory bases (Jakobson, Fant, and Halle, 1951; Singh, 1974) were chosen by Miller and Nicely for predicting the perceptual confusions of consonants. The main questions asked in this experiment were:

1. How well does this feature system explain the confusions of consonants?
2. Does each of these five features transmit equal amounts of information?
3. Are these five features independent of each other?

Figure 5-1 shows the effects of six S/N ratios (abscissa) on the rate of information (ordinate) for the five features and the phoneme. The features nasality and voicing show greater strengths (represented by greater amount of information transmission) than the features duration, frication, and place of articulation. Information rate of the composite channel (phoneme) is placed between these two sets of groups for features.

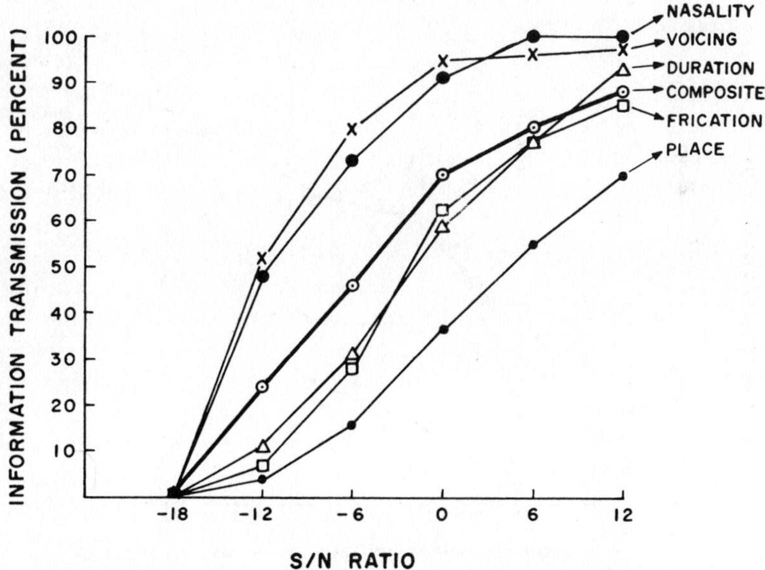

Figure 5-1. Information transmission for nasality, voicing, duration, composite, frication, and place as a function of six S/N ratios. (Data plotted from Miller and Nicely, 1955.)

The results of lowpass and highpass filter conditions are shown in Figures 5-2 and 5-3, respectively. These figures reveal that the features nasality, voicing, and frication had a higher rate of information under the lowpass conditions while the features duration and place of articulation had a higher rate of information in the highpass filter conditions.

Figure 5-4 shows the comparison of the crossover points of the five different features and the composite channel. In this figure, the crossover point for frication is at 750 Hz (4A); for place of articulation at 1,900 Hz (4B); for duration at 2,500 Hz (4C); for composite transmission at 1,250 Hz (4D); for nasality at 450 Hz (4E); and for voicing at 500 Hz (4F). Thus, the crossover points for nasality, voicing, and frication are below and for place and duration are above the crossover point for composite channel.

The results of the Miller and Nicely experiment showed that the different features did not hold similar ranks in speech perception. The

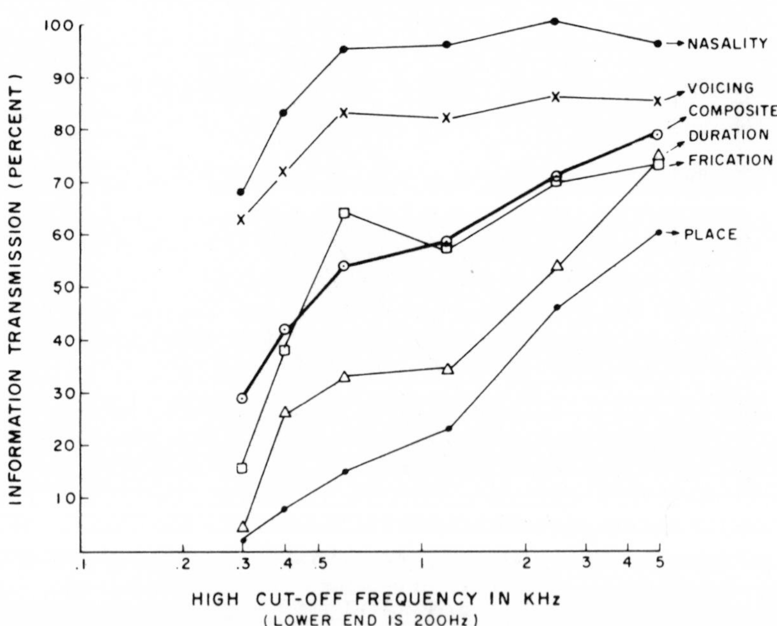

Figure 5-2. Information transmission for nasality, voicing, composite, duration, frication, and place as a function of six lowpass bandwidths. (Data plotted from Miller and Nicely, 1955.)

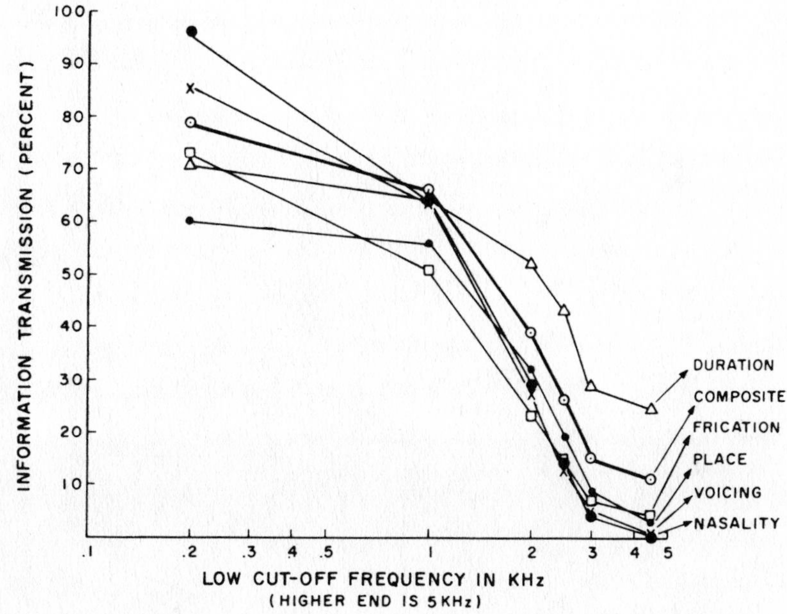

Figure 5-3. Information transmission for duration, composite, frication, place, voicing, and nasality as a function of six highpass bandwidths. (Data plotted from Miller and Nicely, 1955.)

rank order of the features was: 1) nasality (62%), 2) voicing (59%), 3) duration (41%), 4) frication (40%), and 5) place of articulation (27%). More importantly, the lowpass and highpass filters and the different levels of noise affected these features differently.

Singh and Black (1966) In the Singh and Black (1966) experiment the one-language hypothesis of Miller and Nicely was extended to a cross-language experiment. The speakers and listeners of Hindi, English, Arabic, and Japanese spoke and identified an identical set of 26 consonants in the contexts of two vowels. The purposes of the experiment were to establish a common set of parameters or features across the four languages and to investigate the universal application of a selected group of consonant features in speech perception. The quantitative method utilized in this study was the same as described in Miller and Nicely (1955). The Miller and Nicely feature system was extended from five to seven distinctive features for accommodating the distinctions of a larger set of consonants. The object was to find the rank order of the strengths of the features in the error responses of the listeners and their similarity in the different language groups.

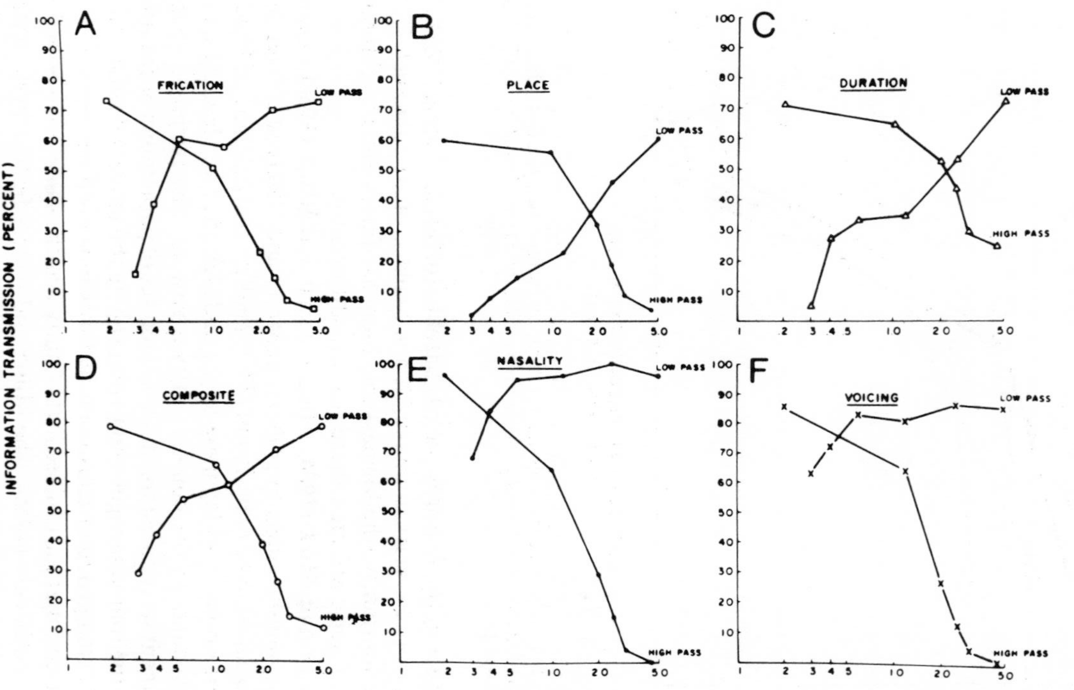

Figure 5-4. Low- and highpass crossover points for information transmission values frication (*A*), place of articulation (*B*), duration (*C*), composite (*D*), nasality (*E*), and voicing (*F*).

The percentage of information transmission in the 16 speaking/listening conditions is shown in Table 5-1. The single rank order in this study was obtained for the four listening groups: 1) nasality, 2) place, 3) liquid, 4) voicing, 5) duration, 6) frication, and 7) aspiration. Such perceptual consistencies on the level of distinctive articulatory features among 16 speaker/listener conditions of four distant languages seem to support the hypothesis of language universals or, more specifically, a universal phonetic theory.

There is general agreement between the rank ordering of features in the experiments of Singh and Black and of Miller and Nicely. However, the feature place of articulation fared far better in the Singh and Black experiment.

Singh (1966) The Singh (1966) experiment included the investigation of the effects of acoustic and linguistic distortions by using speakers and listeners of Hindi and English and by systematically distorting the phonemes on the frequency and time continua. Instead of utilizing consonants of broad phonetic categories, only stops were included in this experiment. The objectives were: 1) to test the effects of filtering and temporally segmenting speech on the intelligibility of plosive consonants as spoken and heard by native speakers of Hindi and English, 2) to determine the predictability of information transmission when three features rather than five were used to describe 12 stops, 3) to ascertain the extent of the preservation of distinctive features in the error responses, and 4) to note subjects' agreements in the responses to the plosives of the two languages.

Six plosive consonants were temporally truncated at 20, 40, 60, 80, 100, and 120 msec, and subsequently passed through a variety of bandpass filters, resulting in a total of 4,320 stimuli for the 10 listening subjects of each of the two languages.

The analysis of the results of the confusion matrices derived from the 10 listeners of each language draws heavily on a quantitative procedure originally used by Miller and Nicely and subsequently adopted in the cross-linguistic study of Singh and Black. Figure 5-5 depicts the performance of the speakers and listeners of Hindi and Figure 5-6 shows the performance of speakers and listeners of English. Both of these figures show the rate of information transmission for the features voicing and place as a function of higher cutoff frequencies. The lower end of the bandwidths in these conditions was fixed at 106, 212, 425, and 850 Hz. A comparison of these figures shows opposite tendencies for the features place and voicing. Place seemed to preserve better than voicing for the speakers and listeners

Table 5-1. Percentage of information transmitted in bits per stimulus for all features and for each feature separately

Condition	All	Voicing	Nasality	Aspiration	Friction	Place	Duration	Liquid
Hindi-Hindi	75.27	60.83	89.89	44.14	54.42	78.35	52.88	54.07
Hindi-English	69.80	50.62	94.94	41.80	52.59	76.29	42.25	61.23
Hindi-Arabic	70.04	67.18	93.43	29.59	57.47	76.29	41.94	85.08
Hindi-Japanese	68.10	75.20	94.94	14.55	12.00	72.68	40.27	66.80
Rank order		4	1	7	6	2	5	3
English-Hindi	64.72	34.06	100.00	26.38	25.22	68.04	36.77	39.16
English-English	75.44	62.70	95.20	28.36	58.90	77.31	54.25	85.28
English-Arabic	72.65	63.43	93.68	34.89	55.64	73.20	54.56	73.95
English-Japanese	71.78	33.53	100.00	17.50	45.67	79.38	40.73	68.98
Rank order		4	1	7	6	2	5	3
Arabic-Hindi	64.74	43.85	86.61	26.26	27.26	71.13	38.30	51.09
Arabic-English	70.53	57.80	64.14	41.30	54.83	71.65	46.50	68.19
Arabic-Arabic	73.42	48.95	97.47	34.03	43.94	76.80	50.76	86.28
Arabic-Japanese	66.68	63.74	95.20	25.03	39.06	71.65	40.27	65.20
Rank order		4	1	7	6	2	5	3
Japanese-Hindi	61.34	44.06	97.47	23.18	21.36	67.53	33.89	47.31
Japanese-English	68.65	52.91	100.00	16.89	44.35	69.59	44.68	54.27
Japanese-Arabic	62.87	50.62	94.44	57.58	31.94	65.98	40.42	62.42
Japanese-Japanese	68.04	73.53	97.47	13.07	47.81	78.35	43.00	66.80
Rank order		4	1	7	6	2	5	3
Overall average (rank order)		4	1	7	6	2	5	3

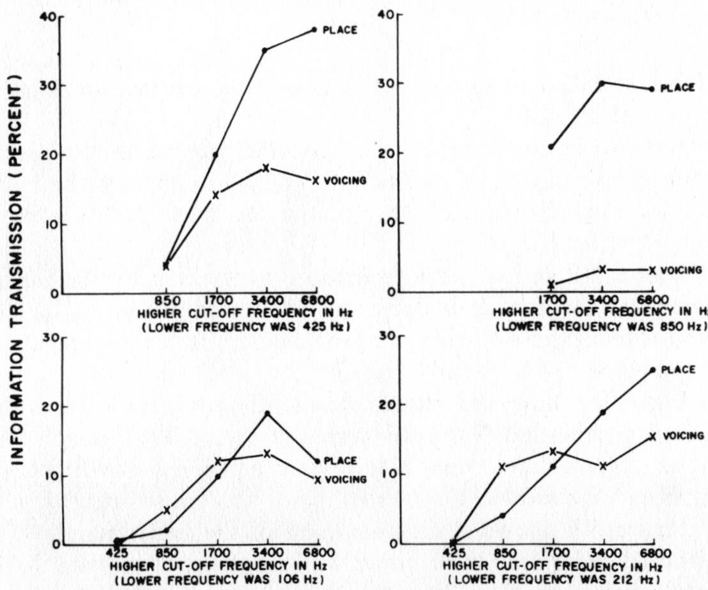

Figure 5-5. Information transmission for place and voicing as a function of fixed lower cutoff frequencies at 106, 212, 425, and 850 Hz. The higher cutoff frequencies were arranged in one-octave steps. The speakers and listeners were Hindi. (Based on Singh, 1966.)

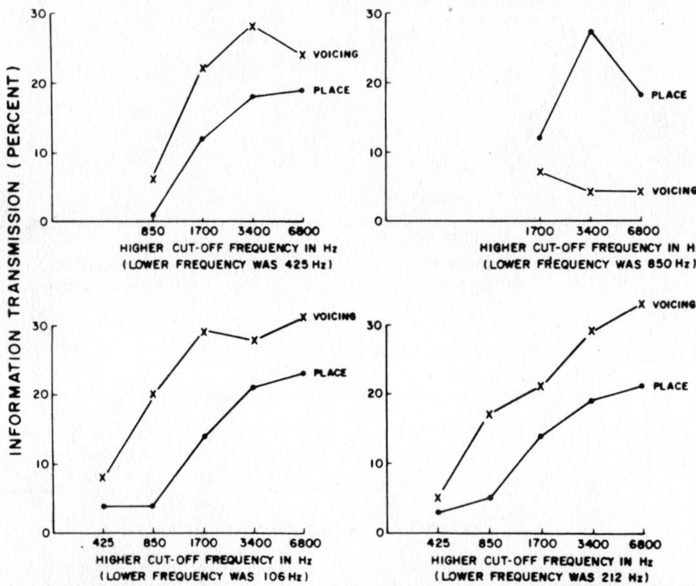

Figure 5-6. Information transmission for place and voicing as a function of fixed lower cutoff frequencies at 106, 212, 425, and 850 Hz. The higher cutoff frequencies were arranged in one-octave steps. The speakers and listeners were English. (Based on Singh, 1966.)

of Hindi, while voicing did better than place for the speakers and listeners of English.

It therefore seems that the voicing and place dichotomy is, to a certain extent, language dependent. Voicing dominates the feature place for English whereas place dominates the feature voicing for Hindi.

Figure 5-7 shows the information transmitted by the features voicing and place of articulation as a function of the six levels of temporal truncations. Again, the language-dependent bases for voicing and place can be clearly seen.

Figure 5-8 shows the comparison of different specifications of the place of articulation feature in terms of the order in which Hindi bilabial, alveolar, and velar places were perceived as a function of frequency bandwidths. The bilabial place was the strongest feature.

Figure 5-9 shows the comparison of the performance of the bilabial, alveolar, and velar places as a function of temporal distinctions ranging from 20 to 120 msec of truncations. For both languages,

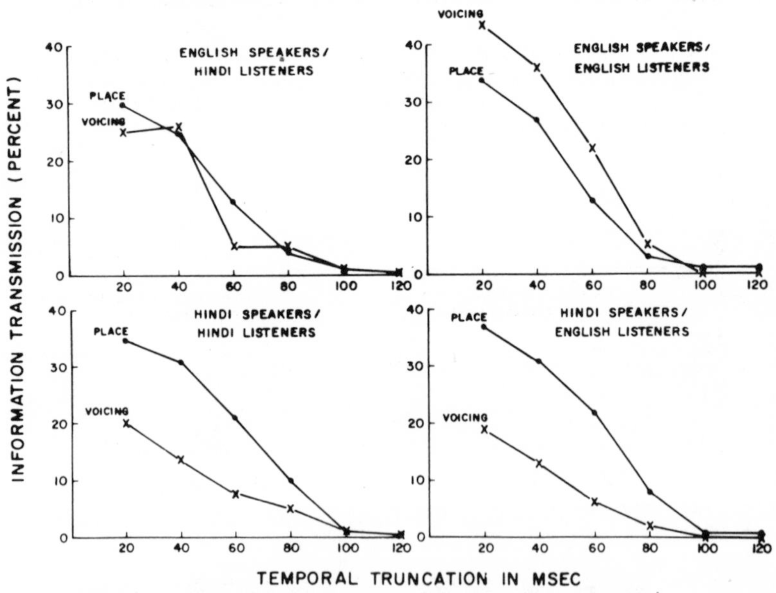

Figure 5-7. Information transmission for voicing and place for the four speaking/listening language groups as a function of six different durations of transaction. (Based on Singh, 1966.)

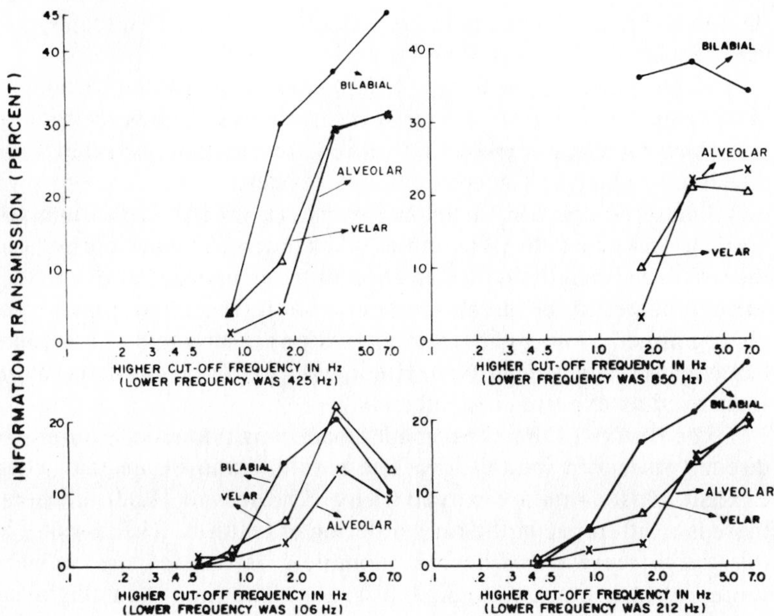

Figure 5-8. Information transmission for bilabial, alveolar, and velar places as a function of fixed lower cutoff frequencies at 106, 212, 425, and 850 Hz. The higher cut-off frequencies were arranged in one-octave steps. The speakers and listeners were Hindi. (Based on Singh, 1966.)

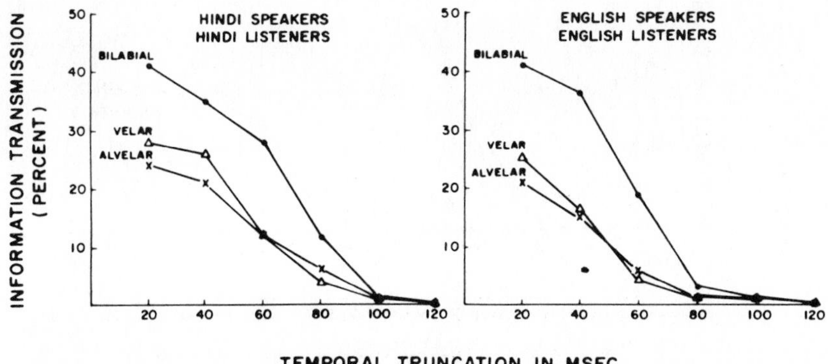

Figure 5-9. Information transmission for bilabial, velar, and alveolar places for Hindi speakers and listeners and English speakers and listeners as a function of six different durations of truncation. (Based on Singh, 1966.)

the bilabial place carried greater amounts of information than either the alveolar or velar places.

Singh (1970a) The Singh (1970a) study investigated the effects of 22 temporally truncated English consonants on the perception of six arbitrarily chosen phonetic features. The features selected were affrication, plosive, voiced, voiceless, nasality, and frication. Two male speakers, one Hindi and one English, recorded 22 consonants of English prevocalically. The initial and relatively longer portions of the syllables (including the transition of the consonant to the vowel) were truncated at the threshold of perception. The gated stimuli were photographed from an oscilloscope for measurements. Listeners from the two language groups, Hindi and English (32 in each group), were used as experimental subjects.

The results of the experiment concerning phonetic features are directly shown in Figure 5-10. The results demonstrate that when English consonants are perceived by English and Hindi listeners, there is a difference in the rank ordering of features. The abscissa in this figure represents selected phonetic features and the ordinate represents the time-to-intelligibility ratio. The time-to-intelligibility ratio was computed by dividing the critical time factor for a feature by

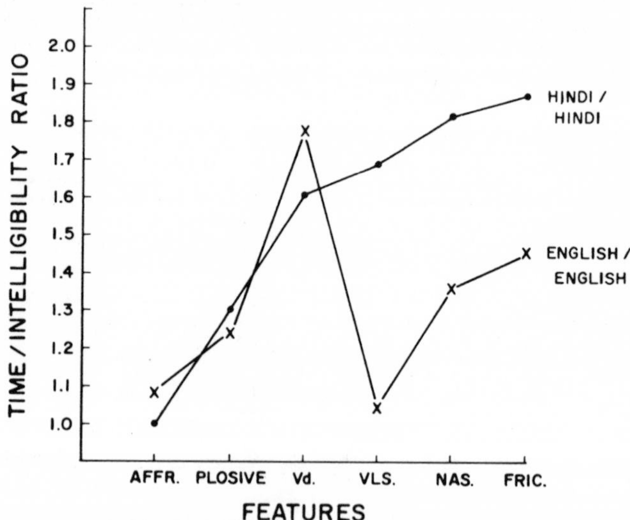

Figure 5-10. Time-to-intelligibility ratio for six features involving Hindi and English speakers and listeners. This ratio was obtained by dividing the smallest amount of time needed for the identification of a consonant by the percentage of identification score associated with it. (Based on Singh, 1970a.)

the number of correct responses (an average for listeners of a language group). The smaller the time-to-intelligibility ratio, the stronger the feature. Figure 5-10 further shows that for both language groups the feature affrication was one of the strongest features. Frication and nasality were weaker features when the temporal factor was the source of distortion. The maximal discrepancies between the two languages existed for the voiceless consonants.

Wickelgren (1966) Wickelgren (1966) investigated the applications of alternative distinctive feature systems in predicting errors in short-term memory for consonants. He compared three distinctive feature systems: Miller and Nicely (1955), Halle (1964), and Wickelgren (1966). The basic assumption underlying the prediction of short-term memory errors by distinctive features is that both perception and short-term memory utilize a similar set of parameters for encoding phonemes. Wickelgren tested the hypothesis that short-term memory errors or intrusion errors in recall are committed not on an all-or-none basis but on a componential basis.

The study included two groups of consonants, one group consisting of the same 16 consonants used by Miller and Nicely and the other group consisting of all 22 consonants of English occurring at the initial position of a syllable. All syllables were of the consonant-vowel (CV) type, and the vowel in each case was /a/.

The main results pertaining to the short-term memory intrusions (recall of a different consonant from the one the subject heard and wrote down) can be summarized by presenting the total percentage of correct feature recall computed for each of the three feature systems. Because the features voicing and nasality had identical specifications in all three feature systems, they resulted in identical feature recall value for each system: voicing 64% and nasality 56%. The remaining three features of the Miller and Nicely system, five features of the Halle system, and two features of the Wickelgren system were the basis for the comparison of the feature systems. Recall of features in the incorrect phonemic intrusions for the Miller and Nicely feature system was 64%, the Halle system 60%, and for the Wickelgren system 74%. Wickelgren concluded that:

> the accuracy of each of the three feature systems is consistently and significantly above chance, indicating that intrusion errors in short-term memory tend to have distinctive features in common with the presented consonant [and that] consonants are *not* remembered in an all-or-none manner. Some of the features of a consonant can be recalled when others cannot, producing a systematic tendency for the errors in short-

> term recall to have distinctive features in common with the correct consonant. This suggests that recall of a consonant means recall of a set of features that defines that consonant in memory, and each feature is recalled at least semi-independently of the other features (p. 397).

It is obvious in this instance, then, that the Wickelgren feature system was a better predictor of the short-term memory intrusions than the Halle and the Miller and Nicely feature systems. The significance of this difference was tested by the chi-square method, and it was found that the Wickelgren system was significantly more accurate than the Miller and Nicely feature system (at the 0.02 level; $\chi^2 = 21.3$).

Singh (1970b) Three different sets of features—Singh and Black (1966), Halle (1964), and Wickelgren (1966)—were compared by Singh (1970b) to investigate which system more closely approximated the judged similarities of English consonants spoken and heard by Hindi and English speakers. The consonants were judged in five S/N ratio conditions and four signal level conditions in both initial and final syllabic positions. The main difference between this experiment and that of Wickelgren's is that Wickelgren's observations were intrusions in recall whereas observations in this study were a measure of similarity judgments, namely, the triadic comparison (ABX).

All responses of the distortion conditions were pooled for distinctive feature analysis. Rank correlations were obtained between the listener's judgment of similarity and the three distinctive feature systems independently. There were eight response matrices, 22 consonants, and three distinctive feature matrices, resulting in a total of 528 rank correlations. One-half of these correlations were found significant at the 0.05 level. A comparison of the consonants in prevocalic and postvocalic contexts showed that 59% of the correlations were significant when judged in the prevocalic position and 43% of the correlations were significant when judged in the postvocalic position. A greater number of rank correlations were significant in the listening mode (60%) than in the speaking mode (42%), implying that the auditory responses were predicted more reliably than the productive responses. An additional comparison of the three feature systems showed that the extension of the Miller and Nicely system by Singh and Black resulted in the largest number (61%) of significant correlations, the Halle system resulted in the second largest number (51%) of significant correlations, and the Wickelgren system resulted in the smallest number (41%) of significant correlations.

The above findings do differ from those of Wickelgren. It may be recalled that Wickelgren reported that his system demonstrated maximal accuracy (73%) when compared with the feature systems of Miller and Nicely and of Halle. The basis for the differing results may be attributable to the different data collection methods involved in the Wickelgren study and the Singh (1970b) study. The responses elicited in the short-term memory and the similarity judgment paradigms yield different preferences for the features.

Ahmed and Agrawal (1969) In the Ahmed and Agrawal (1969) study, 29 consonants of Hindi at the initial place of a CVC syllable and 31 at the final place were combined with 10 nondiphthongized vowels of Hindi to comprise the test material used for listening. A total of 870 different nonsense CVC syllables were recorded for presentation by one female and two males. No syllable had the same consonant in the initial and final positions. The syllables were randomized and presented to six male listeners in nine sessions.

Information transmission was obtained from two confusion matrices, one involving the 29 consonants in the initial position of a syllable and one involving the 31 consonants at the final position of the syllable. A feature system somewhat similar to the one used by Singh and Black was used to describe the Hindi consonants.

Although the results showed some consistencies existing across positions between rank orders of the importance of features (from most important to least important), there were some crucial differences. The two features nasality and aspiration demonstrated the most pronounced differences between their ranks at the initial and final positions. Both of these features fared well at the initial positions, with second and third rankings, respectively. However, they were extremely weak at the final positions, with rankings of seven and nine. Place of articulation was another unstable feature. It ranked eighth at the initial position and fifth at the final position. This finding further indicated that, contrary to the tendencies of nasality and aspiration, place is a stronger feature at the final position of a syllable.

A comparison of one Miller and Nicely condition (+12 dB S/N ratio in the 200- to 6,500-Hz bandwidth) and one Singh and Black condition (Hindi speakers/Hindi listeners) with the results of the present experiment revealed a great number of discrepancies. It should be noted, however, that these three experiments were conducted in entirely different experimental conditions. Some of the outcomes of the comparisons are as follows:

1. Initial position data in the Ahmed and Agrawal study agreed well with the data of Miller and Nicely.
2. There was no correlation between the data of Singh and Black and of Ahmed and Agrawal.

3. There was no correlation between ranks at the initial and final positions of a syllable in the Ahmed and Agrawal data.
4. The rank order of features of consonants depended strongly on the consonant's position in a syllable. A particular example of this finding is the differences observed for the feature place in the experiments of Miller and Nicely, Singh and Black, and Ahmed and Agrawal. In Miller and Nicely's study the feature place was found to be the most difficult to hear correctly. The feature place, however, was found to be highly intelligible for various language groups in Singh and Black's experiments. Place was further observed to be more difficult to hear in the initial position rather than in the final position, as found in the Ahmed and Agrawal study.

Gupta, Agrawal, and Ahmed (1969) The only procedural difference between the earliest study by Ahmed and Agrawal and this experiment (Gupta, Agrawal, and Ahmed, 1969) is this study's utilization of distorted syllables by clipping the peaks of the signal. According to Gupta, Agrawal, and Ahmed (p. 770), the purposes of this experiment were:

1. To determine the effect of clipping on the intelligibility of both the individual consonants and their features.
2. To compare the rank order of the feature system of clipped speech with that of normal speech.
3. To correlate the different amounts of information given by initial consonants and final consonants, and to note the difference in consonant perception for these two positions.

The effect of clipping was computed by subtracting the information content of a feature in the clipped speech from that in normal speech. In the initial position of the syllable, maximal distortion occurred for the place of articulation (30.85%) whereas minimal distortion occurred for the feature affrication (4.32%). The rank order of features, in initial position, from the most to the least susceptible to clipping distortion, was: place (30.85%), nasality (20.49%), liquid (17.99%), continuancy (17.33%), aspiration (9.74%), voicing (9.52%), frication (5.00%), and affrication (4.32%). In the final position of the syllable, the greatest amount of clipping effect was seen for the feature nasality, whereas the smallest amount was observed for affrication. The rank order of features, in final position from most to least susceptible to the clipping distortion, was: nasality (30.36%), frication (26.79%), place (25.01%), liquid (23.83%), voicing (22.46%), flapped liquid (21.09%), aspiration (19.55%), continuancy (19.12%), and affrication (10.47%). Affrication was the strongest feature in the clipping condition whereas nasality and place were the weaker features.

By utilizing the criterion of the differential effect of clipping, a comparison was made of the initial and final positions. Figure 5-11 represents plottings of the effect of clipping on the eight different features at both initial and final positions of a syllable. Two clear conclusions can be drawn on the basis of this figure. First, there is generally a greater clipping effect on the final consonants than there is on the initial consonants. Second, place of articulation is the only feature that shows a reverse tendency to the above conclusion.

Figure 5-11 also shows the maximal difference of the clipping effect for the feature frication. The effect of clipping for the initial and final consonants was correlated with a rank order correlation of 0.52. This correlation was not found to be significant. However, the rank correlation between the initial consonants of normal speech and the initial consonants of clipped speech was significant (0.78). Also found to be significant (0.88) was the rank correlation between the final

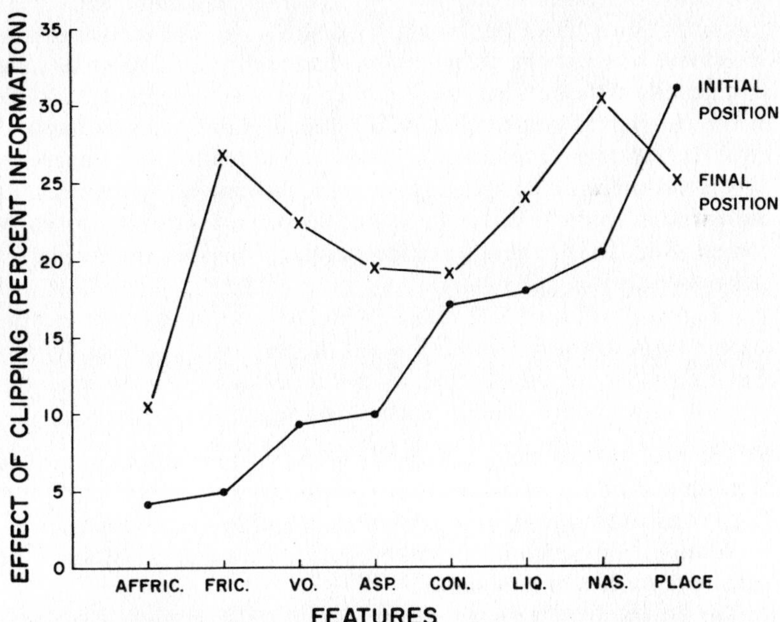

Figure 5-11. Effect of clipping on eight different features in the initial and final consonantal positions. The effect of clipping is the difference of transmitted information in the undistorted and clipped conditions. (Based on Gupta, Agrawal, and Ahmed, 1969, and Ahmed and Agrawal, 1969.)

consonants of normal speech and the final consonants of clipped speech. These two significant correlations seem to indicate that, in spite of the clipping distortions, the position of the consonants in a syllable plays a significant role. This finding is further substantiated by the lack of correlation between the initial and final consonants in normal speech (0.21) and between the initial and final consonants in clipped speech (0.05).

Singh (1971) The purpose of the Singh (1971) investigation was to find whether the minimally distinct consonant pairs have different perceptual strengths and whether these strengths change under different S/N ratios and filter conditions. The minimally distinct pairs of consonants defined by the feature systems of Miller and Nicely and Halle were included in this experiment. Each stimulus-response unit consisted of a triad (ABX) of CV syllables. The listeners were asked to judge whether the stimulus was more similar to the first or the second stimulus-response choice.

In the six experimental conditions, 846 similarity judgments were obtained from three groups of 33 subjects. Chi-square tests were computed for each of the minimally distinct pairs of consonants to determine whether the responses associated with these pairs were significantly different from one another. Fifty-nine percent (501/846) of the chi-square values showed significant differences at the 0.01 level. It was therefore concluded that a one-feature difference between consonants led most judges to perceive one of the members as more similar to the stimulus in 59% of the pairs. However, in 41% of comparisons, the one-feature difference did not lead to any consistent perception for the subjects.

Figures 5-12 and 5-13 show the relative mean strength on the ordinate and distortion conditions on the abscissa. In these figures, the higher the mean perceptual distance value, the greater the strength of a feature. These figures also depict the following:

1. The distinguishing characteristics of the voicing feature improved in noise and deteriorated in quiet conditions.
2. The feature frication improved in quiet and deteriorated in noise.
3. When in competition with other features in quiet conditions, the voicing feature was less stable.
4. The noise characteristics of frication were easily lost in the experimental noise.
5. Duration as an added cue (e.g., /s, z, ʃ, ʒ/) did improve the distinguishing characteristics of some of the fricatives.

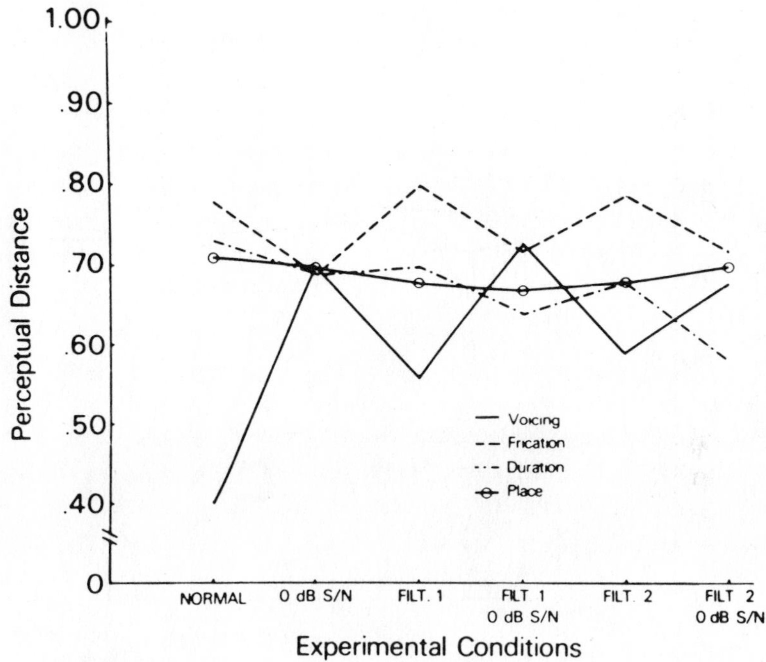

Figure 5-12. Perceptual strength of the features voicing, frication, duration, and place as a function of six listening conditions. The greater the distance, the greater the strength. (From Singh, 1971.)

6. Nasality contained the maximal distinction in all six conditions of listening.
7. Nasality, liquid, and glide were minimally affected by the filtering and noise conditions.

Wang and Bilger (1973) The focal points of the Wang and Bilger (1973) study include: 1) which features best accounted for performance in a consonant discrimination task, and 2) whether the same features were best throughout a variety of contexts and listening conditions. The assumption was that, if it is possible to determine the exact nature of the perceptual features and if these features are invariant, then these features may be considered natural perceptual categories.

Twenty-four initial and 19 final consonants of English (from a total list of 25 consonants) were combined with the three vowels /i, a, u/. Four syllable sets (CV_1, VC_1, CV_2, and VC_2) were constructed

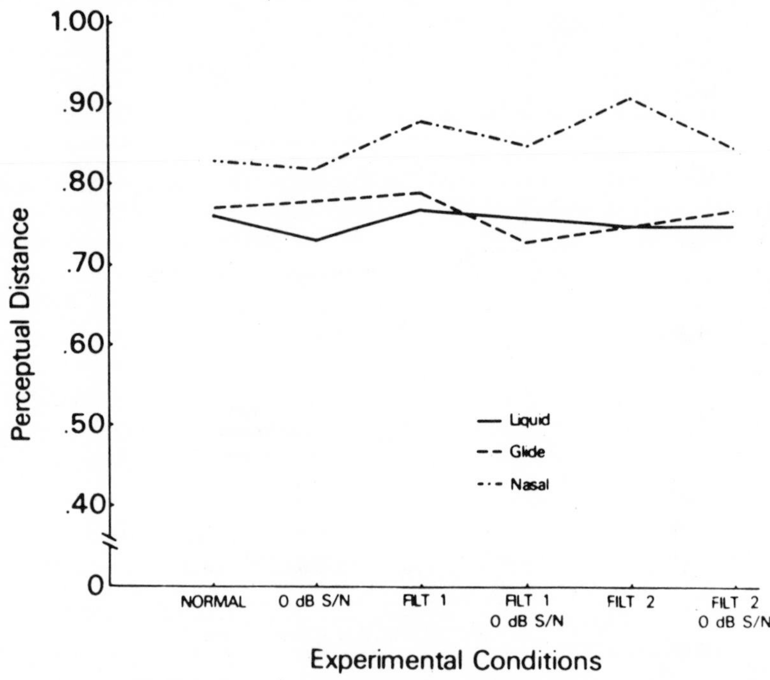

Figure 5-13. Perceptual strength of the features liquid, glide, and nasality as a function of six listening conditions. The greater the distance, the greater the strength. (From Singh, 1971.)

from these initial and final consonants, each consisting of 16 syllables. Each of the four sets of stimuli was heard in six S/N ratio conditions and four level conditions. There were three replications of each of the 24 (six S/N ratios × four signal levels) experimental conditions, yielding a total of 72 experimental conditions. In the control experiment there was no noise introduced. Different reductions of the signal level were utilized to determine intelligibility. Six subjects were used as listeners.

In the distinctive feature analysis of the experiment's results, an inventory of 19 grossly overlapping features was used: 1) vocalic, 2) consonantal, 3) high, 4) low, 5) back, 6) coronal, 7) anterior, 8) voicing, 9) nasality, 10) continuancy, 11) stridency, 12) round, 13) frication, 14) duration, 15) place (Miller and Nicely), 16) place (Singh and Black), 17) place (Wickelgren), 18) sibilancy, and 19) openness. These features include a complete set of five feature systems, namely, the systems of Miller and Nicely (1955), Singh and Black (1966), Wickelgren (1966), Chomsky and Halle (1968), and Singh, Woods, and Becker (1972).

The results showed that for the CV_1 syllable set, only four of the 12 features tested were consistently found to contribute to discrimination performance. These four features were voicing, sibilancy, high-anterior, and frication. With the exception of voicing, a lack of consistency was apparent regarding the importance of features for the VC_1 syllable set. There was considerable agreement in terms of the relative importance of features across the six listening conditions in the CV_2 syllable set. The five features that were consistently identified in the iteration program were: vocalic, nasality, round, high, and voicing. Because of the nature of consonants in the syllable sets CV_1 and CV_2, the first three of these features—vocalic, nasality, and round—were not represented. Thus, the only two features that could be tested across the syllable sets CV_1 and CV_2 were high-anterior and voicing. These two features were consistently important to the syllable set. The consistently important features for the VC_2 syllable set were voicing, nasality, continuancy-open, and frication.

The broad categories of features investigated in this experiment can be viewed as falling within three general groups. First, nasality, voicing, and roundness were perceptually important wherever they occurred. Second, stridency and low showed opposite tendencies, since they were not found to be significant in any of the conditions. Third, the remainder of the distinctive features were only of variable importance.

Wang and Bilger also examined comparable data from two earlier studies, Miller and Nicely (1955) and Singh and Black (1966). Eleven of the 19 features listed in the Wang and Bilger study were used as criteria to compare the data of Miller and Nicely with the data of Wang and Bilger. A very close agreement was found between the results of Wang and Bilger's CV_1 syllable set and Miller and Nicely's 200- to 6,500-Hz bandwidth in +12 dB S/N ratio condition. The features that were identified as being important in both analyses were voicing, sibilancy, frication, and place. Because nasality was not included in the Wang and Bilger CV_1 syllable set, it could not be used in a direct comparison. Nasality, however, was the best perceived feature in Wang and Bilger's other sets where nasal consonants were included. Sixteen of the 19 features in the Wang and Bilger study were used as criteria in a comparison between the Singh and Black data and the Wang and Bilger data. Nasality, vocalic, voicing, and place of articulation were distinguished in both experiments. The features frication and sibilancy were both identified in only one analysis.

Figure 5-14 shows a plotting of the features (nasality, sibilancy, anterior (place), continuancy (frication), and voicing as a function of the six S/N ratios. Consistent with earlier results (Singh, 1971) it can be seen that the feature nasality was strong across most conditions. Voicing was strong only in conditions of severe noise, whereas sibilancy and place were weak in severe noise and strong in less severe noise conditions. The feature continuancy was weak across all conditions.

On the basis of the statistical analysis of these data, Wang and Bilger concluded that the distinctive articulatory and/or phonological features of consonants account for most of the transmitted information (more than 90%) in a stimulus-response condition. For example, the Singh and Black feature system accounts for 94% of the information. However, beyond certain points there were alternative features that could explain the remaining small amount of variance. Wang and

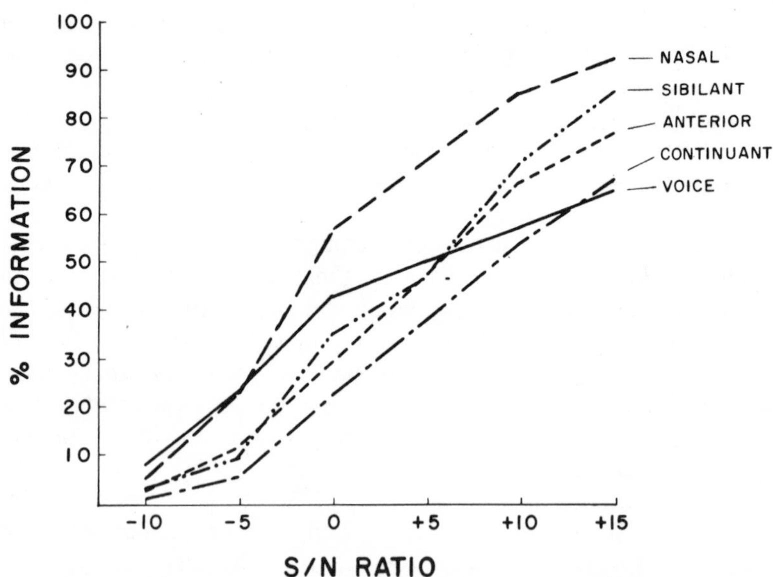

Figure 5-14. Information transmitted for the features nasality, sibilancy, anterior, continuancy, and voicing as a function of six S/N ratios. (Based on Wang and Bilger, 1973.)

Bilger concluded that there is little support for the hypothesis that natural features or feature systems exist. This conclusion was based on their findings that several feature systems accounted equally for the transmitted information and that there were no particular features or feature systems better than others across varying conditions and syllable sets.

Prediction of Different Sets of Perceptual Responses by a Number of Feature Systems

A phoneme is considered an abstract entity that man acquires at an early age. The phonetic and auditory processes are man's efforts to manifest the abstract in speaking and listening behaviors. The purpose of the experiments under the present heading is to approximate most closely the "true" or the "abstract" location of the phoneme in the repertoire of a native speaker. The different data collection methods may require slightly altered perceptual strategies on the part of the subject. However, all methods attempt to determine the closest approximation to the "true" location of a phoneme in the speaker's perceptual repertoire. The data collected by Singh, Woods, and Becker (1972) and Singh and Becker (1972) revealed the common perceptual properties of phonemes across three data collection methods.

Singh, Woods, and Becker (1972) The similarities of 22 English consonants were judged by three different methods of comparing stimuli. These judgments were analyzed mainly by multidimensional analysis. This technique of analyzing perceptual responses has proved extremely promising (Danhauer and Singh, 1975a,b). The commonly retrieved distinctive features of speech perception were: 1) place (front/back), 2) nasal, 3) sibilant, 4) voice, and 5) plosive. These features correlated highly with several of the phonologically derived features in the Chomsky and Halle (1968) feature system.

Singh and Becker (1972) In the Singh and Becker (1972) experiment, four feature systems were used to predict perceptual judgments using three psychological methods: 1) seven-point scaling (SF), 2) magnitude estimation (ME), and 3) triadic comparison (ABX). The feature systems examined were: 1) Miller and Nicely (1955), 2) Singh and Black (1966), 3) Wickelgren (1966), and 4) Chomsky and Halle (1968). Multiple correlation of the three data collection methods and the four feature systems was all found to be statistically significant at the 0.001 level of confidence. It was noted, however, that none of the correlations was higher than 0.663.

Role of Distinctive Features in Dichotic Processing of the Phoneme

It has been shown that speech sounds are perceived by a language-dominant left hemisphere. Because the distinctive features are considered the basic component of a phoneme, it is important to know: 1) whether all features have significant tendencies toward the dominant hemisphere, and 2) whether some features show a greater amount of dominance than others.

In general, dichotic listening tasks require the subjects either to identify stimuli or to make judgments from simultaneous presentation of two stimuli, one in the left ear and the other in the right ear. Different studies have utilized varying stimuli, procedures, and analyses.

Studdert-Kennedy and Shankweiler (1970) In the Studdert-Kennedy and Shankweiler (1970) experiment, four dichotic tests, two for consonants and two for vowels, were constructed involving six stop consonants and the six vowels /i, e, æ, a, o, u/. For analysis, the stop consonants were elaborated in terms of the feature voicing and place of articulation. Each consonant was considered either voiced or voiceless and also as having one of the three places of articulation: labiality, alveolarity, and velarity. The rate of percentage of information transmitted by each of these features for both the right and left ear transmission systems was determined. The comparison for the feature voicing showed an information value of 49% for the right ear and 31% for the left ear. Comparison for the feature place of articulation showed a right ear information transmission value of 32% and a left ear value of only 22%. Even though both features demonstrated feature lateralization, it is evident that voicing was a stronger feature than place. On the basis of the experimental findings, it was concluded that independent features underlie consonant lateralization. A comparison of the laterality effect on feature perception in the initial and final contexts showed that there was more prominent right ear advantage for both features for the initial consonants of a syllable than for the final consonants.

Cole and Scott (1972) The study by Cole and Scott (1972) investigated subjects' judgments of same/different for a syllable pair, and the reaction time required for such judgments. Eight consonants, specifying the features grave, diffuse, strident, nasal, continuant, and voiced, were chosen for testing. All consonants were paired with the vowel /a/. In addition to a number of identical trials in both left and right ears, each of the other seven sounds was paired twice (once in each ear) with a given sound. The main finding of this experiment was a plotting of reaction time on the ordinate and the number of distinctive feature differences on the abscissa, as shown in Figure 5-15. In this figure, zero difference implies that the stimuli in both ears were the same. The results demonstrate that distinctive features of vowels and consonants were valid criteria to predict their discrimination when the criterion of reaction time was used. The reaction time was greatest when the pairs of syllables were most similar, whereas the reaction time was smallest when the pairs of syllables were most dissimilar. The similarity was determined by counting the distinctive feature difference between the two pairs. The orderly effect of feature difference on reaction time was significantly different (F, 7.07; $df = 5$; $p < 0.001$) when the pairs of phonemes appeared simultaneously in both ears and when subjects were performing a discrimination task.

Blumstein and Cooper (1972) In the Blumstein and Cooper (1972) study, six English plosives were dichotically discriminated in one test and dichotically identified in another. The distinctive feature

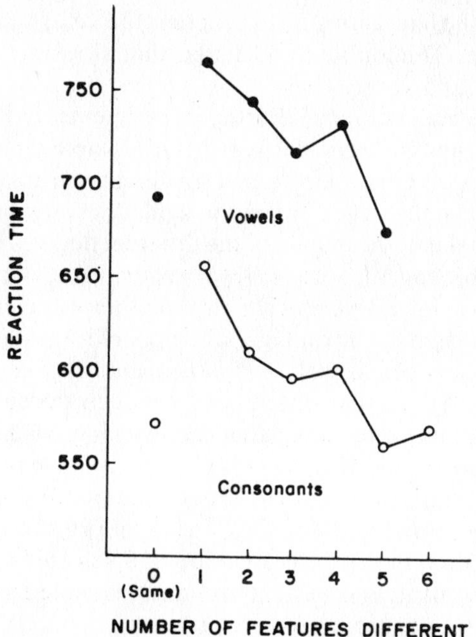

Figure 5-15. Reaction time values associated with feature differences between pairs of consonants and pairs of vowels. The reaction times of the same pairs of consonants and vowels are also shown. (From Cole and Scott, 1972.)

analysis of the confusions of consonants was reported for both discrimination (judgment of same/different) and identification tasks. The distinctive feature principle was operative in the discrimination task as evidenced by the better discrimination score when the pairs of consonants differed by two features instead of by one feature. However, in the identification task, the scores were poorer when the consonants differed by two features as compared to one feature. This unexpected result was explained by proposing that the identification task required encoding of the message in short-term memory, whereas the discrimination task did not require such encoding. The feature differences in the identification task had to be stored in short-term memory as well as be processed for discrimination. This additional processing, it is hypothesized, "loaded" the system and resulted in poorer scores.

Day and Vigorito (1972) In a dichotic task reported by Day and Vigorito (1972), temporal order judgments of synthetic syllables were investigated for plosives, liquid, and vowel categories. It was reported that the stops showed the right ear advantage (liquid was neutral regarding the laterality effect), whereas the vowel showed the left ear advantage. The authors concluded that stops are encoded more than liquids and vowels are.

Crystal and House (in Press) Earlier experiments by Blumstein and Cooper (1972) and by Day and Vigorito (1972) were replicated by Crystal and House (in press) with signal modifications aimed at elucidating the role of signal level. When the syllables were masked by speech-shaped maskers, the impact of the different degrees of encoding reported by Day and Vigorito (1972) was minimized. Crystal and House equated the signal levels of the different phonetic categories and minimized the right ear advantage. Their conclusion was that the major difference between vowels and consonants is their inherent level of intensity. Perceptual differences between consonant and vowel may be minimized by equalizing the listening conditions.

Blumstein, Tartter, and Michael (1973) The Blumstein, Tartter, and Michael (1973) study investigated the perceptual reality of selected distinctive features in dichotic listening. The authors utilized only the manner of articulation in their investigation of a selected number of English stop, continuant, and nasal consonants presented to subjects for identification. The consonants were presented in the CV context, and only one- and two-feature different contrasts were tested. An example of a one-feature contrast is nasality (/ba/ in one ear, /ma/ in the other). An example of a two-feature contrast is nasality and place

(/ba/ in one ear, /za/ in the other). Analysis of the results revealed the following particulars:

1. The overall identification of consonants was significantly greater in the right ear.
2. The manner features fricative and stop were identified a significantly greater number of times in the right ear than in the left ear.
3. The manner feature nasality showed no significant difference between the right and left ear identifications.

A POSTERIORI STUDIES

The a priori feature systems lack the flexibility of adding a "new" feature or eliminating a "known" feature, depending on what the perceiver's actual response strategies were. These systems also lack the essential assumption of any scientific investigation, that of testing the relevance of the known attributes without eliminating the possibility of discovering the unknown. The a priori feature systems were used only because there was no suitable direct method for determining the speech perception parameters in an a posteriori fashion.

The following discussion reports perceptual features of phonemes proposed a posteriorily. The data analyzed by this method were obtained from different stimulus sets, data collection methods, speaking/listening conditions, response modalities, ages, language backgrounds, and hearing disorders. The central theme of this discussion is that, in spite of the above described diversities, speech perception research shows a strong tendency of invariance for certain perceptual features.

The work of experimenters whose goal was to retrieve a posteriori features of phonemes can be divided into three groups: 1) those who worked with factor analysis and some other less defined spatial model; 2) those who worked with a better defined metric and nonmetric multidimensional scaling analysis of the proximity data; and 3) those who worked with a multidimensional scaling analysis technique found to be more suitable for speech perception research, e.g., INDSCAL (individual differences scaling).

Retrieval of Distinctive Features by Factor Analysis and Other Spatially Less Defined Methods

Klatt (1968) In a reanalysis of Wickelgren's (1966) short-term memory data, Klatt (1968) used a similarity metric to determine : 1) the statistical level of significance of a feature in predicting the errors, 2) the inadequacy of any feature system so far utilized to explain the errors, and 3) the degree of independence of the features. Most of Klatt's results were based on the computation of a measure of duration from the total number of cross-set confusions (Dev (Ncs)). This measure is computed from binary confusion tables involving a given number of predetermined features. A value of Dev (Ncs) computed to be greater than 3.0 was interpreted as highly significant. The distinctive features selected for evaluation with the associated Dev (Ncs) were: voiced (3.55), long fricative (8.27), sonorant (6.61), continuant (4.63), strident (6.70), anterior (1.89), coronal (2.24), nasal (2.01), and consonantal (1.58). When these Dev (Ncs) were conditionally computed, only the following Dev (Ncs) were found to be significant: voiced (3.55), long fricative (8.26), sonorant (4.97), and continuant (3.44). The conditional Dev (Ncs) of a feature is determined by considering the existence of the feature preceding it. Therefore, the binary features in the data with a confidence level greater than 0.99 were voiced, long fricative, sonorant, and continuant.

A further analysis by Klatt investigated whether the features that had been arbitrarily selected by Wickelgren were significant in accounting for the variance in Wickelgren's data. In addition to the features listed, the feature sibilancy was included for computation of the Dev (Ncs) value. The resulting figure was 3.57, which is significant at > 0.99. This finding indicates that the sibilancy grouping, although not included in the initial test of the features, constitutes an important classification strategy for describing short-term memory errors.

Black (1970) Black (1970) used factor analysis to group consonants of English without an a priori assumption that the groupings would correspond with the categories plosive, fricative, lateral, glide, etc., or with systems of distinctive features. Twenty-four consonants were paired with five vowels and judged for degree of similarity. Factor analysis (rotated by VARIMAX routine) was used to isolate 12 factors. Only the first four factors were such that more than one consonant had contrastively high factor loadings. The first factor was nasality, with the loading of 0.91 for /m/ and /n/ each. The second factor was the slit fricative, with positive factor loadings for /θ/, /ð/, /f/, and /v/ of 0.89, 0.69, 0.94, and 0.64, respectively. The third factor was a long duration or grooved fricative with high factor loadings of 0.86, 0.87, and 0.93 for /s/, /z/, and /ʒ/, respectively, and a moderate factor loading of 0.45 for /ʃ/. The remainder of the factors in this study isolated one consonant per factor; this is not considered an elegant assignment.

Wilson (1963) Wilson (1963) reanalyzed the data of Miller and Nicely (1955) by a multidimensional procedure. He used an earlier version of Shepard's (1962) multidimensional scaling (MDS) technique, along with his own adaptation of that technique. Wilson reported clear interpretation of the two features, voicing and nasality, in the Miller and Nicely data. Some less clear interpretations possible were the features sibilancy and continuancy. The feature place of articulation did not show any strength. Furthermore, the feature sonorancy was not obtained because sonorants were not included in the stimuli.

Johnson (1967) Johnson (1967) tested the applicability of his model against the data of Miller and Nicely (1955) using a hierarchical clustering scheme. This method converts the perceived distances between stimuli into a series of rank-ordered diameters. With this method, the diameter values located along the vertical dimension can be utilized to provide certain well bifurcated clusters that are arbitrarily used to define the number of important groupings in the data. The important clusters reported by Johnson from the Miller and Nicely data were nasality, voicing, and sibilancy.

Shepard (1972) In a reanalysis of the Miller and Nicely data by the Shepard technique of scaling, Shepard (1972) reported the features voicing and nasality in a two-dimensional solution. This solution accounted for 99.4% of the variance in the data. The two-dimensional solution presented by Shepard actually can be reinterpreted by an additional feature, sibilancy, which separates /s, ʃ, z, ʒ/ from all other consonants.

Peters (1963) Peters (1963) primarily focused on the spatial representation of the 16 English consonants whose interpoint distances were secured by feeding the psychologically obtained proximities among consonants to an earlier multidimensional analysis technique (Torgerson, 1958). Perceptual judgments were made on a seven-point scale. Peters reported the recovery of the major perceptual features voicing, manner, and place. However, a reexamination of the spatial representations of his stimuli reveals that the feature manner could be elaborated in terms of nasality, sibilancy, and continuancy.

Shepard (1972) Shepard (1972) reanalyzed Peters' data using his own multidimensional scaling analysis technique and reported the recovery of the perceptual features voicing and nasality. A reexamination of Shepard's reanalysis reveals that, in addition to the two reported features, nasality and voicing, the feature sibilancy also can be shown to exist on one of the two dimensions reported.

Graham and House (1971) In the Graham and House (1971) study, 4.5-year-old children performed same/different judgments on pairs of consonants presented at the word-medial positions. Graham and House used the Shepard-Kruskal method of nonmetric multidimensional scaling to determine the dimensionality and the features of consonant perception. They failed to obtain significantly relevant perceptual correlates to the expected phonetic features for the 4.5-year-old children. They did report a tendency of these children to utilize the features nasality, continuancy, and sonorancy. However, there was a lack of clear interpretation of the results for all these features.

Singh, Woods, and Tishman (1972) Singh, Woods, and Tishman (1972) reanalyzed the Graham and House data with an underlying metric assumption for describing judgments of either Euclidean or City-Block phonemic pairs (see Singh, Woods, and Becker, 1972). The perceptual judgments of children analyzed with these underlying assumptions yielded results compatible with the phonological competence of 4.5-year-old children and consistent with the adult model. The 16 consonants were found to have been perceived by these children in a two-dimensional space with nasals, sibilants, continuants, and sonorants each forming distinct perceptual groups.

Jeter and Singh (1972) Jeter and Singh (1972) constructed 336 triads from eight prevocalic English consonants and presented them to 60 judges, 30 of whom compared them for auditory similarities and 30 of whom made judgments of visual similarities. All of these judgments were made in an ABX paradigm. The Shepard-Kruskal method was used to analyze the judgments. A plotting of Kruskal's (1964a, 1964b) measure of stress for both auditory and visual perception indicated that these triadic judgments regarding the eight consonants were made in a three-dimensional space. The concept of stress, in multidimensional scaling, refers to the "goodness of fit" of the actual data compared to the predicted data. The lower the stress, the better the fit. The visual data have a lower stress, hence a better fit, than the auditory data. The spatial representation of the graphemes in a three-dimensional space revealed that the subjects used vertical-rounded, vertical-crossed, and angular categories exclusively when making visual judgments. The spatial representation of the phonemes in a three-dimensional space revealed that the features voicing and sibilancy were used exclusively when making auditory judgments. It was interesting, however, to note that the features place of articulation and stop/continuant manner were commonly recovered in both visual and auditory modalities. On the basis of the above findings, two sets of overlapping feature systems, one for the eight graphemes and another for the eight phonemes, were proposed. When these features were used to predict the MDS dimensions, the multiple R was 0.809 for the visual space and 0.677 for the auditory space.

Retrieval of Distinctive Features by INDSCAL

Like other multidimensional scaling analyses, one primary objective of the INDSCAL model is to convert psychological proximity of stimulus × response to a set of dimension coordinates.

Carroll and Chang's INDSCAL (1970) is uniquely suitable for providing a spatial representation of the speech stimuli in a number of dimensionalities. These dimensions, or axes, are all assumed to be orthogonal. Thus, all interpretive angles are in a 90-degree relationship. The dimensions in perceptual space may be weighted according to their contributions, in the subject's estimation, of the proximity between stimuli. Additionally, the individual subject's private space or the individual subject's contribution to the perceptual dimensions obtained for the group is also available for scrutiny in this method.

Wish (1970) Wish (1970) reanalyzed the Miller and Nicely (1955) data and reported a much greater number of dimensions than reported earlier by Shepard. Wish found the features nasality, voicing, sibilancy, continuancy, and the second formant transition. A comparison of INDSCAL analysis of these data via Wish's results with those of the MDS analyses (of the same data) via Wilson's, Shepard's, and Johnson's results, shows that a higher and more elaborate structure can be obtained by the INDSCAL analysis. This was not feasible by earlier multidimensional analysis procedures.

Pruzansky (1970) Pruzansky (1970) used 16 consonants, the same ones used by Miller and Nicely, and obtained similarity judgments via a sorting device. She subjected the psychological judgments to INDSCAL analysis and obtained the features nasality, sibilancy, continuancy, and place of articulation.

Singh, Woods, and Becker (1972) The Singh, Woods, and Becker (1972) study involved three data collection methods, SF, ME, and ABX, a large number of subjects, and 22 initial consonants. Through the use of both the Shepard-Kruskal MDS and the INDSCAL procedures, Singh, Woods, and Becker investigated appropriate perceptual dimensionality for diadic and triadic comparisons, the weights of the perceptual dimensions under various data collection methods, and the comparison of the features obtained under the a posteriori methods of analysis (INDSCAL) with that of an a priori feature system. Figures 5-16 and 5-17 show the spatial representations of four of the five dimensions (the fifth dimension was nasality). These figures show front/back, sibilant/nonsibilant, plosive/nonplosive, and voiced/voiceless divisions. The voiced nonplosive consonants can be further subdivided into sonorant /m, l, w, r, j/ and nonsonorant /v, ð, z, dʒ/. The phoneme /n/ is an exception to this classification.

Figure 5-18 shows the manner in which the three data collection methods commonly weight the five dimensions. The abscissa repre-

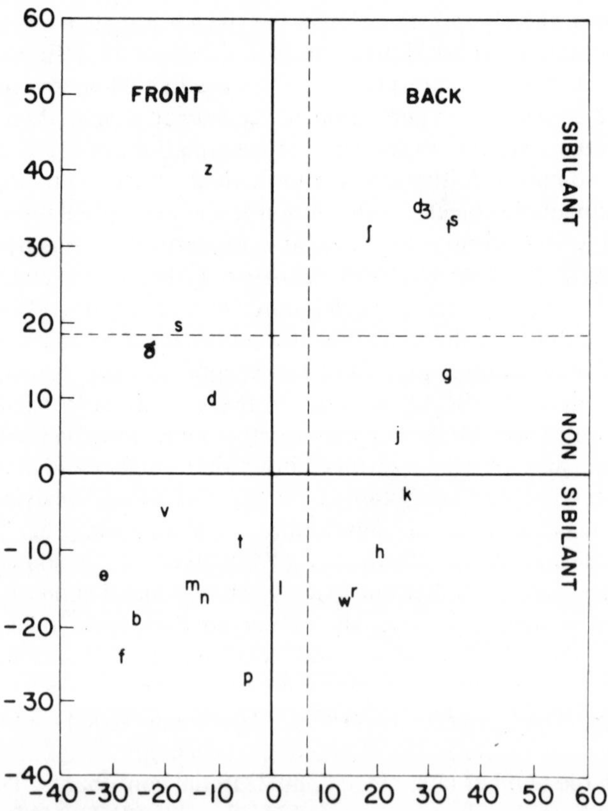

Figure 5-16. Plotting of dimensions 1 and 2 of the five-dimensional INDSCAL configurations. Dimension 1 separates sibilant from nonsibilant, and dimension 2 separates front from back place. (From Singh, Woods, and Becker, 1972.)

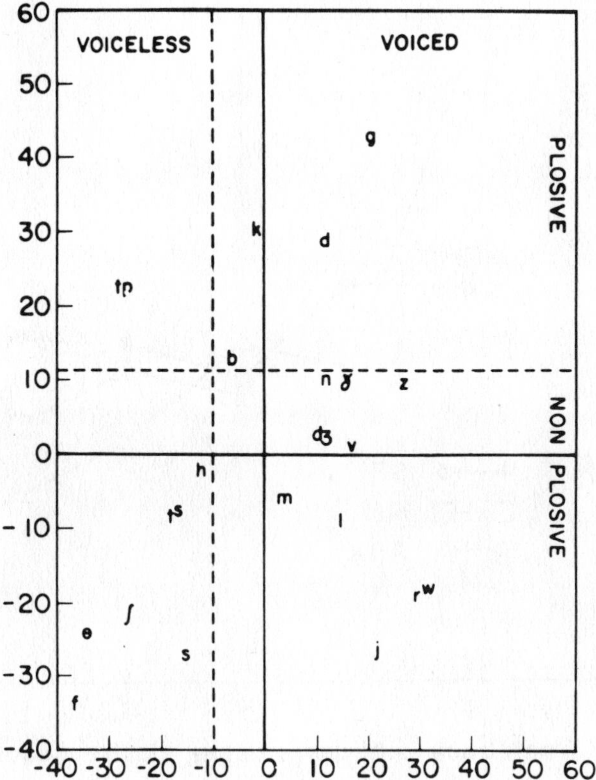

Figure 5-17. Plotting of dimensions 3 and 4 of the five-dimensional INDSCAL configurations. Dimension 3 separates plosive from nonplosive, and dimension 4 separates voiceless from voiced. (From Singh, Woods, and Becker, 1972.)

sents the five dimensions, each representing a perceptual feature. The ordinate depicts the weighting or contribution of each of these dimensions toward the total explained variance. The figure reveals similar weighting tendencies for the diadic method. The triadic method, however, weights place of articulation considerably more than any other feature. The features sibilancy and place are strong for all the three conditions, whereas the feature nasality is weak. It may be noted that the weakness of nasality and the strength of place as an outcome of psychological judgments directly contradict the rank order of features in the Miller and Nicely experiment. These reversals may be attributed to the methods of collecting responses and the experimental conditions.

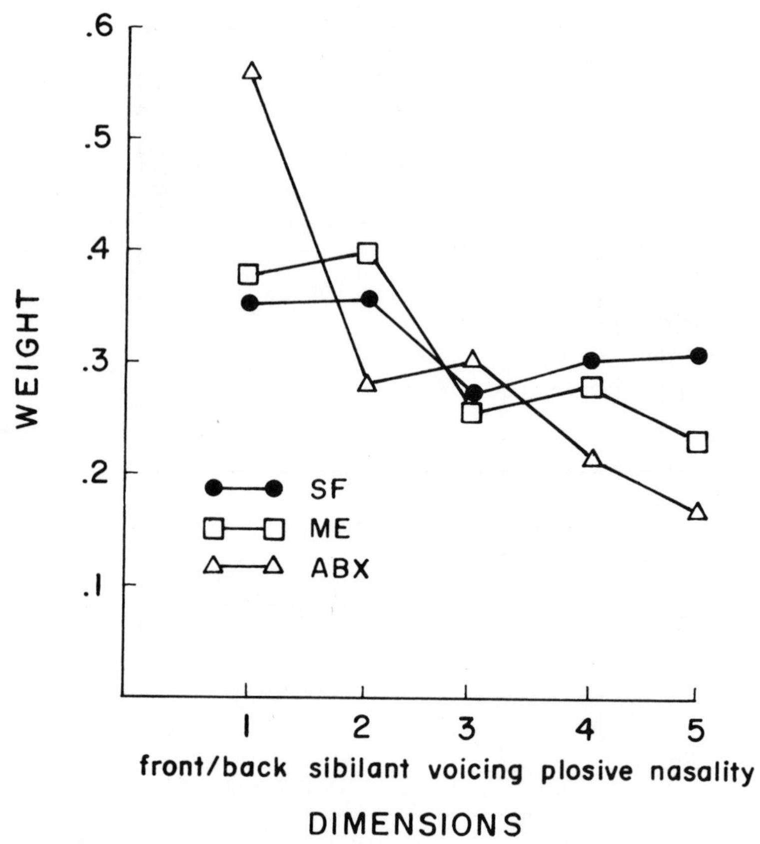

Figure 5-18. Weighting of dimensions and their feature interpretations by three different methods treated as three individual subjects in the INDSCAL analysis. (From Singh, Woods, and Becker, 1972.)

Singh and Singh (1972a) Three sets of perceptual responses to Hindi consonants by Hindi speakers and listeners were analyzed in the Singh and Singh (1972) study. One set of responses was obtained for 28 initial consonants at five S/N ratio conditions from 10 Hindi listeners. The other two sets of responses were obtained for 29 initial and final consonants in the peak-clipped (Gupta, Agrawal, and Ahmed, 1969) and in the undistorted listening (Ahmed and Agrawal, 1969) conditions.

Initial Hindi Consonants in Noise Subjects' confusions for the 28 consonants were obtained in five S/N ratio conditions (6 dB, 3 dB, 0 dB, −3 dB, and −6 dB). For the purpose of obtaining common perceptual space across these conditions, in one of the analyses the data for the 10 judges were pooled for each of the five conditions separately, and the conditions themselves were treated as individual subjects. Before the subjects' perceptual confusions were analyzed by INDSCAL, they were analyzed by MDS (Kruskal, 1964) in one- to six-dimensional spaces. Such a two-step multidimensional scaling strategy facilitates the INDSCAL analysis by reducing the number of iterations it may require for meeting the criterion for solution. Three features—voicing, aspiration, and sibilancy—were obtained on three of the four dimensions of the INDSCAL analysis, while the results in the higher dimensions (five to seven) indicated the presence of some interacting features. Figure 5-19 shows the plotting of two of the four

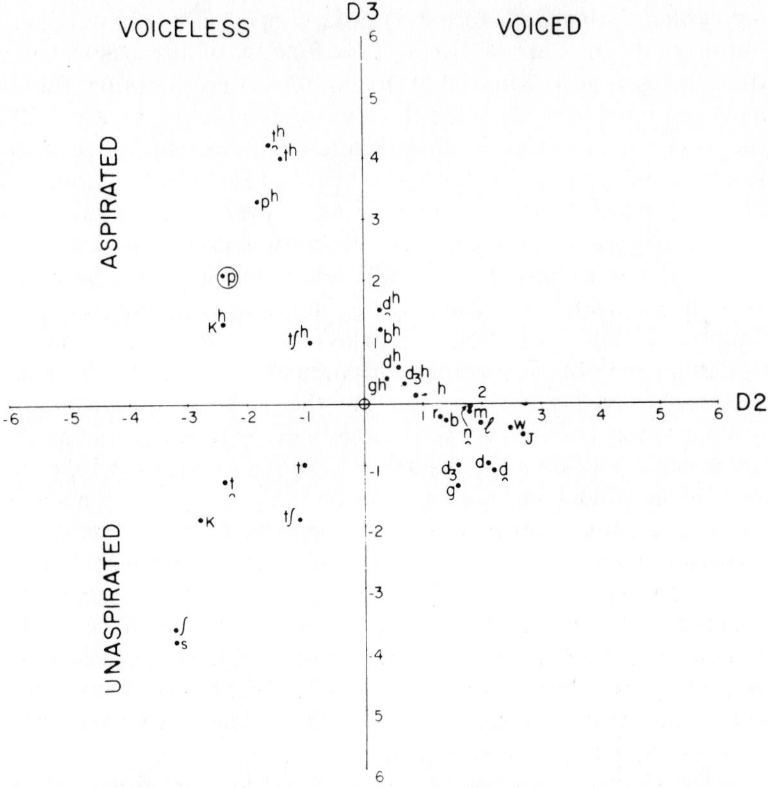

Figure 5-19. Plotting of dimensions 1 and 2 in a four-dimensional space of INDSCAL analysis of 29 Hindi consonants. (Based on Singh and Singh, 1972.)

INDSCAL dimensions. These dimensions were interpreted by the features voicing (/h/ in Hindi is voiced) and aspiration. It may be noted that recovery of the INDSCAL dimensions is constrained by the assumption of the orthogonality or the independence of the coordinate systems. The phonologically distinctive features, voicing and aspiration, therefore, were perceptually utilized independently by the listeners of the Hindi language.

Initial and Final Hindi Consonants in Undistorted and Clipped Conditions Four confusion matrices, two involving initial and final consonants in the undistorted condition and two involving initial and final consonants in the clipped condition, were, again, first analyzed by MDS in one- to six-dimensional spaces. The MDS distances in the six-dimensional spaces were analyzed by INDSCAL, treating as individual subjects each of the following four conditions: 1) initial undistorted, 2) final undistorted, 3) initial clipped, and 4) final clipped. Plotting of the measure of "stress" as a function of dimensions in the MDS analysis shows a much lower value along the dimensions for the unclipped conditions than for the clipped conditions (Figure 5-20). The lower stress value is an indication of better fit between the observed and expected distances in the Kruskal method of scaling. It may be noted that the effect of clipping on the magnitude of fit was substantially greater for the postvocalic consonants than it was for the prevocalic consonants. In the undistorted condition, however, the position of consonants did not seem to influence stress differentially. Figures 5-21 and 5-22 show the recovery of the features voicing, aspiration, and sibilancy as common parameters utilized by the Hindi listeners across the two positions for the peak-clipped and undistorted listening conditions. The recovery of the features voicing and aspiration in four-dimensional space, again, showed their independence in the Hindi language. In dimensions higher than four, no clear indication of any other features was apparent. Some indications of interaction of the sonorancy, nasality, and place features were found.

Walden and Montgomery (1973) Walden and Montgomery (1973) obtained similarity judgments for diads of 20 English consonants by 18 subjects, six with normal hearing, six with mild hearing losses, and six with severe hearing losses. Using INDSCAL they found four-dimensional space for these groups with the features voicing, sibilancy, continuancy, and sonorancy.

Mitchell and Singh (1974) Mitchell and Singh (1974) collected perceptual judgments via ABX on 16 English consonants embedded

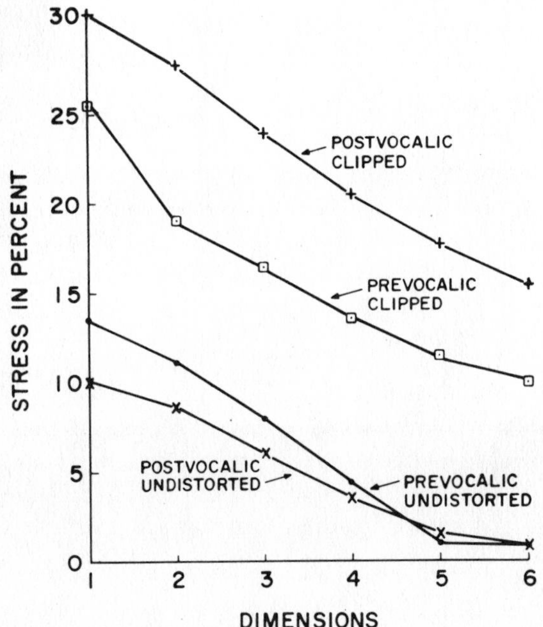

Figure 5-20. Stress as a function of dimensions for the clipped and undistorted listening conditions in pre- and postvocalic contexts. (Reanalysis of data from Gupta, Agrawal, and Ahmed, 1969, and Ahmed and Agrawal, 1969, by Singh and Singh, 1972a).

in a declarative sentence. These sentences were presented triadically in one condition of quiet and two conditions of noise. The INDSCAL solutions were considered in a four-dimensional space for the extreme noise condition and in a five-dimensional space for the quieter conditions. The features obtained in the five-dimensional space were nasality, voicing, sibilancy, continuancy, and place. Because no sonorant consonants other than the nasals were included in the stimuli, there was no provision for the feature sonorancy to be retrieved. The conclusion drawn in this experiment was that the perceptual features obtained in isolated syllables of earlier studies exist also in words embedded in a sentence.

Weiner and Singh (1974) Weiner and Singh (1974) analyzed the judgments of same/different and their choice reaction time (CRT) for nine continuant consonants. The CRT values for each pair of the different consonants were analyzed by INDSCAL analysis. A four-

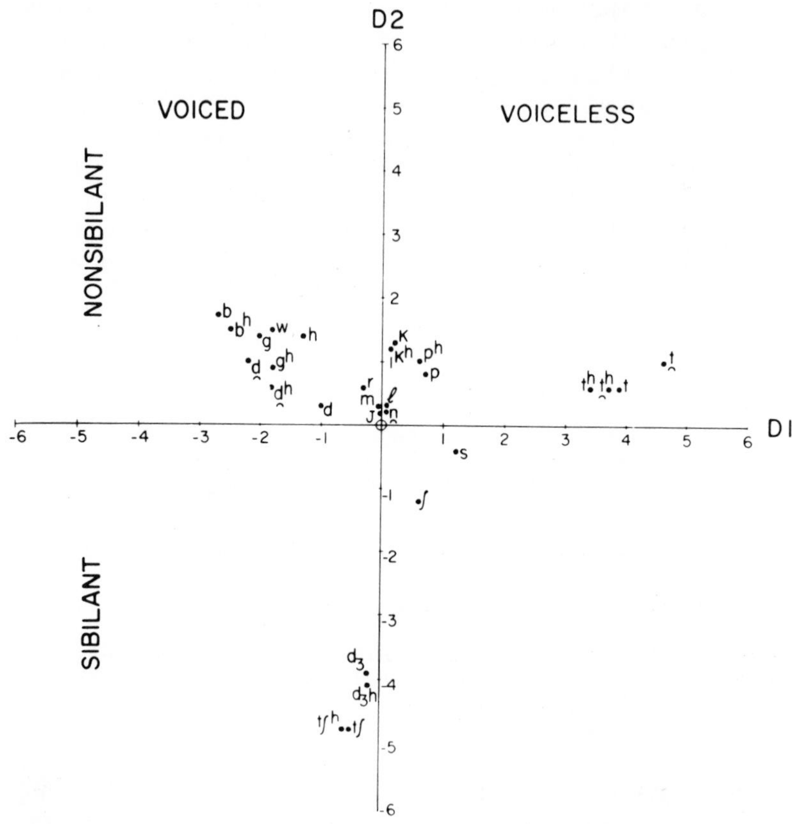

Figure 5-21. Plotting of dimensions 1 and 2 in a four-dimensional space of INDSCAL analysis of 28 Hindi consonants. (Reanalysis of data from Gupta, Agrawal, and Ahmed, 1969, and Ahmed and Agrawal, 1969, by Singh and Singh, 1972a).

dimensional space was considered uniquely appropriate for the CRT measure. These dimensions were interpreted by the features voicing, sibilancy, and two places of articulation. The four-dimensional solution accounted for 72% of the variance in the subjects' judgments. Of the 72%, dimension 1 (voicing) accounted for 24%; dimension 2 (sibilancy) for 19%; dimension 3 (front/back) for 15%; and dimension 4 (palatal) for 14%. These results show that, although it is possible to determine a feature system for a category of phonemes, it is difficult to draw conclusions about the relative weightings of features for that group.

On the basis of the four dimensions recovered in this study, it is assumed that CRT judgments can be used as a criterion for determining phonemic similarity. Figure 5-23 shows CRT as a function of zero-, one-, two-, three-, and four-feature differences. The top curve in Figure 5-23, taken from Chananie and Tikofsky (1969), clearly shows a lack of relationship between CRT and distinctive feature differences. The curve labeled "Weiner and Singh GI" represents the mean CRT's for pairs of consonants representing zero-, one-, two-, three-, and four-feature differences obtained for the same 10 subjects

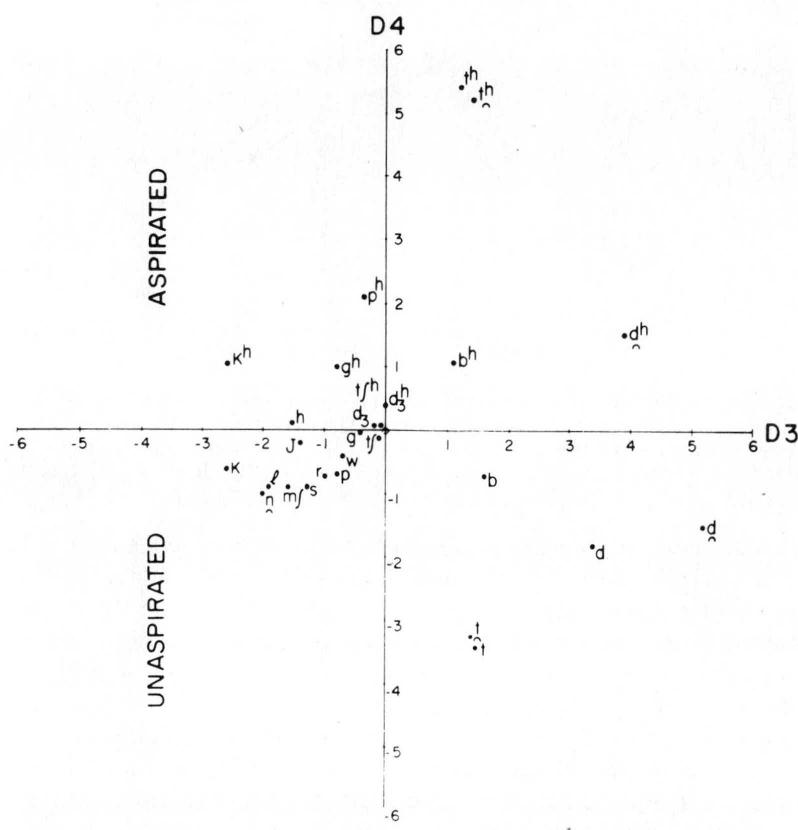

Figure 5-22. Plotting of dimensions 3 and 4 in a four-dimensional space of INDSCAL analysis of 28 Hindi consonants. (Reanalysis of data from Gupta, Agrawal, and Ahmed, 1969, and Ahmed and Agrawal, 1969, by Singh and Singh, 1972a).

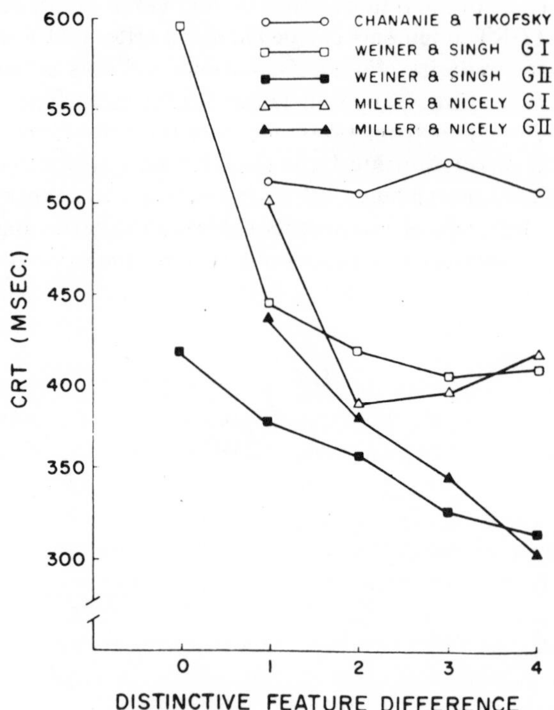

Figure 5-23. Choice reaction time as a function of distinctive features for data collected from groups 1 (G I) and 2 (G II) in the Weiner and Singh (1974) study as compared with a previous study of Chananie and Tikofsky (1969). (From Weiner and Singh, 1974. Copyright 1974 by the American Psychological Association. Reprinted by permission.)

whose judgments were utilized for obtaining the perceptual features. The curve labeled "Weiner and Singh GII" is the outcome of a replication experiment conducted to cross-validate the trend obtained for the first group of subjects. To determine whether these functions showed similar relationships, a comparison of slopes procedure (Dixon and Massey, 1969) was performed. The result was that the two beta coefficients were not different from each other.

A test of the significance of the mean CRT scores associated with the feature differences by a single factor, repeated measures analysis of variance yielded a significant F ratio $(4, 36) = 16.08, p < 0.05$. A Tukey (a) comparison of means (Winer, 1971) showed that CRT values for zero-feature differences were significantly greater than values associated with any other feature difference. In addition, the CRT value associated with a one-feature difference was significantly greater than differences of three and four features.

The curves labeled "Miller and Nicely GI" and "Miller and Nicely GII" are a result of applying Miller and Nicely features, rather than the features obtained from the INDSCAL analysis, to the Weiner and Singh data. The results attributed to the two sets of features were compatible. The difference between the results of the present investigation and those of Chananie and Tikofsky (1969) may be attributed to their level of reaction time, which was considerably higher than the reaction time obtained in the Weiner and Singh (1974) study. Figure 5-23 suggests that the number of features distinguishing one phoneme from another becomes more crucial when the overall magnitude of reaction time is lowered. The magnitude was highest in the Chananie and Tikofsky study, and the number of features played no role. The magnitude was lower in the Weiner and Singh GI, and the slope was not steep. The magnitude was lower in Weiner and Singh GII and Miller and Nicely GII, and the slopes were steepest. Thus, it seems that when extraneous factors contributing to reaction time are minimized, the difference in the number of features begins to play a role.

Danhauer and Singh (1975a) The research by Danhauer and Singh (1975a,b) included three experiments dealing with speech perception by hearing-impaired subjects. The overall goal of these experiments was to determine what features were used by these subjects in their perception of consonantal stimuli. Sixteen English consonants, all voiced/voiceless cognates in English, were judged in the context of a phrase. Three psychological methods, SF, ME, and ABX, were employed for obtaining similarity judgments (Danhauer, 1974). The subjects were three different groups of bilateral sensorineural hearing-impaired individuals. One group of four subjects had a loss of 30 dB or greater at and above 4,000 Hz, the other group had a loss of 30 dB or greater at and above 2,000 Hz, and the third group had a loss of 30 dB or greater at and above 500 Hz. The experimental variables consisted of two conditions, one consistent with the slope of the hearing loss for the particular group and the other a nonfiltered condition.

The similarity judgments made by four subjects in each of the three hearing-impaired groups using the three data collection methods under the filtered and nonfiltered conditions were analyzed by INDSCAL. Within each of the three experiments, this analysis was performed for each of the three data collection methods separately. A common perceptual space was then obtained by combining the three data collection methods.

Features for the 4,000-Hz Group The results of INDSCAL analysis in two- to seven-dimensional spaces revealed that these subjects consistently utilized sibilancy, continuancy, front/back place, and voicing features. In some instances the place feature showed further distinctions of palatal, labial, and dental places.

Features for the 2,000-Hz Group A two- to seven-dimensional INDSCAL analysis showed that, although the feature sibilancy was recovered for the 4,000-Hz group, it was almost never found to exist for the 2,000 Hz. The features retrieved with consistency were plosive, stop/continuant, front/back, and voiceless/voiced.

Features for the 500-Hz Group The commonly retrieved features across the three methods and two conditions for this group were, again, voicing, sibilancy, stop/continuant, and front/back place. The most persistent feature for this group was voicing. For this group, one of the strongly weighted dimensions was most frequently interpreted as sibilancy, continuancy, and plosive on one dimension without violating the assumption of orthogonality in INDSCAL. This is an extremely economic and neat perceptual strategy rarely seen in data obtained from normally hearing subjects in undistorted conditions. The fact that subjects with losses above 500 Hz processed consonants utilizing such high frequency features implies that the phoneme perception by these subjects supersedes the concept of critical frequencies.

Conclusions Three conclusions can be drawn from these three experiments. First, the filtering did not affect either the recovery or the weighting of features in any of the experiments in a predictable fashion. Second, the perceptual features of consonants were recovered by invoking "cues" not directly related to acoustic thresholds, thus making it possible for the subjects with sharp slopes in pure tone sensitivity beyond 500 Hz to be able to utilize features of high frequency characteristics. Third, the perceptual features obtained for these three groups of subjects were similar to the ones reported earlier under conditions of noise (Mitchell and Singh, 1974) and quiet (Singh, Woods, and Becker, 1972). In a CVCV stimulus, the severely hearing-impaired or deaf subjects seem to process vowel information by their residual low frequency hearing (since most hearing losses occur in the high frequency areas and most vowel information is contained in the low frequency areas). The hearing-impaired subjects are usually unable to process consonant information because consonants mostly contain high frequency energies. Consonants, then, are perceived as blanks in the temporal continuum by the hearing-impaired subject. Since consonants are of characteristic lengths, these subjects perform some sort of temporal patterning to detect features. For example, sibilants are typically of greater duration. Voicing information is probably processed by these subjects on the basis of the presence versus absence of low frequency formant characteristics. Most hearing-impaired subjects can hear the low frequency energy component of a voiced consonant. If such perceivable low frequency energy is absent, they deduce a voiceless consonant. In conclusion, severely hearing-impaired and deaf subjects utilize a perceptual strategy different from that of normal subjects yet derive almost a comparable amount of feature information from the minimal cues available to them.

Danhauer and Singh (1975b) Cross-linguistic responses were obtained to CVCV stimuli by severely hard of hearing and profoundly deaf French, American, and Yugoslavian subjects with average pure tone thresholds poorer than 90 dB ISO for frequencies above 1,000 Hz. The responses were analyzed by the INDSCAL procedure. The perceptual features obtained from these subjects were nasality, voicing, sonorancy, sibilancy, and continuancy. Although these are aggregated features for all subjects, the extent of hearing disorders in the above subjects (12 for each language—six hard of hearing and six deaf) was such that, on the basis of pure tone audiograms, it would not be possible to explain the retrieval of some of these features. It is concluded in this study that the perceptual features of phonemes do not depend directly on the decoding of acoustic cues. These features seemed to be entities unto themselves without direct correlations with the acoustic properties of the stimuli and the auditory capacity of the perceiver.

Danhauer and Appel (in Press) The last consonantal study reported in this chapter involves a cross-modality comparison of the perception of consonants. Responses from 24 subjects to the initial consonants of English in visual (print), tactile (vibrations), and visual-tactile modalities were obtained to investigate the retrieval of the perceptual features of the consonants from cues other than those supplied directly by the auditory modality. An INDSCAL analysis of the subjects' confusions revealed that these subjects utilized voicing, sibilancy, continuancy, and labial place features.

Conclusions Although it has been shown that the features nasality, voicing, sibilancy, continuancy, sonorancy, and place seem to have been retrieved consistently, there are still some cases where they have failed to be recovered. Three reasons for such a lack are being posited here. First, the earlier multidimensional studies did not examine high enough dimensionality to obtain all features (Shepard, 1972). Second, a given perceptual feature was too sensitive to a given experimental condition and assumed zero weight because of that condition. Place of articulation, in noise, was such a feature (Mitchell and Singh, 1974; Singh, 1971). Since the majority of the experiments reported here involved noise, either experimentally induced or because of hearing losses, place feature showed extreme weakness. The third reason is that the weakness in the initial structure of the data, attributable to lack of sufficient observations to warrant involvement of all features (in a confusion matrix), was felt to be another reason for the lack of recovery of certain features (Danhauer and Appel, in press).

CONCLUSIONS

Independence of Perceptual Features

The perceptual features appearing persistently in the studies reported in this chapter were voicing, nasality, sibilancy, continuancy, sonorancy, and front/back place. Listeners' performance in utilizing these features in various experimental and listening conditions shows predictable patterns. These features have potentials of being described simultaneously by the selected articulatory and acoustic features. However, while the perceptual features may utilize the articulatory and acoustic properties in manifesting themselves, they are entities into themselves, thereby *superseding* man's possibilities in both the auditory and productive domains. The recovery of high frequency features like place of articulation and sibilancy, perceived by normal subjects and by severely hearing-impaired young adults of several languages (Danhauer and Singh, 1975a,b), demonstrates the independence of features from close auditory ties. The hearing-impaired subjects, whose audiograms show appreciable hearing losses at and above 500 Hz, have the ability to utilize these features in a complex perceptual task (Danhauer and Singh, 1975a, b). These results cannot be explained by a theory of audition.

Similar to the findings that phonemic perception may defy auditory principles, phonemic perception also defies articulatory principles. In a cross-linguistic experiment (Singh and Black, 1966) it has been shown that listeners from Hindi, English, Arabic, and Japanese languages made perceptual errors with sophistication that was not a part of their phonetic repertoire. The perceptual processing of aspiration by the English listeners, liquid/retroflexion by the Japanese listeners, and of a much larger group of fricatives by Hindi listeners, cannot be explained by the phonetic ability of the subjects in these languages. It is concluded, therefore, that like the acoustic parameters the articulatory parameters provide only a manifesting medium for the perceptual processes.

Satisfaction of Certain General Criteria for a Theory

The six perceptual features of consonants found in the a posteriori analyses are essentially similar in nature to the important features in the a priori experiments. The manner in which these features have been recovered seems to satisfy certain broadly accepted criteria for a theory. These criteria may include: 1) simplicity and economy, 2) unambiguity, and 3) potential to explain data. For simplicity, the only classification system of the perceptual features obtained in the a posteriori studies involved was a clear binary division of the phonemic distinctions, disregarding all other details. For economy, in spite of the inherent redundancy in the phonemic system, the obtained dimensionality in these studies was closely tied with the exponents of the binary base. An examination of several independently conducted research studies involving phoneme perception, with varying subjects, conditions, stimuli, speakers, listeners, modalities, deviances, etc., consistently reveals these perceptual features.

chapter 6
Distinctive Features in Vowel Perception

CONTENTS

Hanson (1967)
Pols, Van der Kamp, and Polmp (1969)
Singh and Woods (1971)
Anglin (1971)
Terbeek and Harshman (1971)
Shepard (1972)
Grant (1971)

In order for a theory of speech sounds to be acceptable, it should handle perceptual features of vowels as well as of consonants. Because the consonants and the vowels are not typically represented on a continuum, the features used to describe them are different. All of the studies presented here use a posteriori features of vowel perception.

HANSON (1967)

Hanson (1967) conducted a series of experiments in which he investigated the perceptual similarity of natural and synthesized Swedish vowels. A factor analytic output provided two interpretable dimensions, by F_1 and F_2, that relate to the height and advancement dimensions of the vowel system.

POLS, VAN DER KAMP, AND POLMP (1969)

Pols, Van der Kamp, and Polmp (1969) used a Shepard-Kruskal multidimensional analysis technique to analyze the perceptual output of 11 normalized vowels. Two of the dimensions that accounted for most of the variance in the data were advancement and height.

SINGH AND WOODS (1971)

Singh and Woods (1971) obtained numerical ratings of dissimilarity using 12 isolated American English vowels and analyzed them by means of the Shepard-Kruskal nonmetric procedure of multidimensional scaling. The features were interpreted from a three-dimensional analysis as tongue height, tongue advancement, and retroflexion, although retroflexion distinguished only the vowel /ɝ/. Figure 6-1 shows a plotting of 12 vowels in three-dimensional space. The original set of MDS coordinates for the vowels were rotated with the target configurations of advancement, height, and retroflexion. The placement of vowels on the three perceptual dimensions mirrors the articulatory mapping of English vowels.

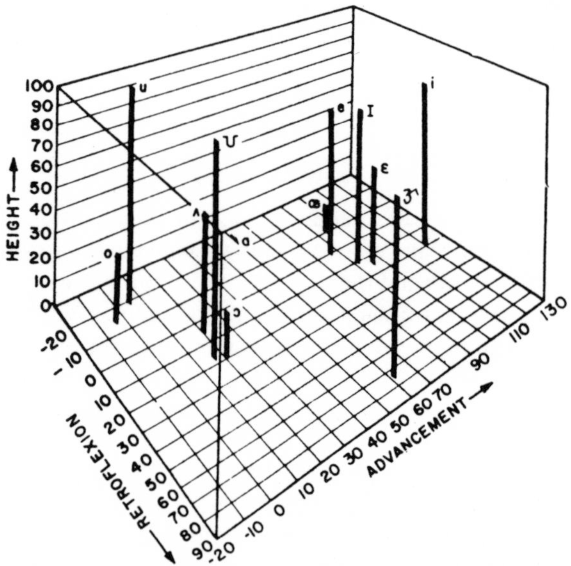

Figure 6-1. Rotation of three-dimensional configuration of MD-SCAL output (From Singh and Woods, 1971.)

ANGLIN (1971)

In a perceptual study of 12 English vowels in the context of meaningful words, Anglin (1971) reported a four-dimensional solution. Figures 6-2 and 6-3 are the plottings of these spaces. Figure 6-2 shows a mirror image of a traditional vowel diagram with advancement inter-

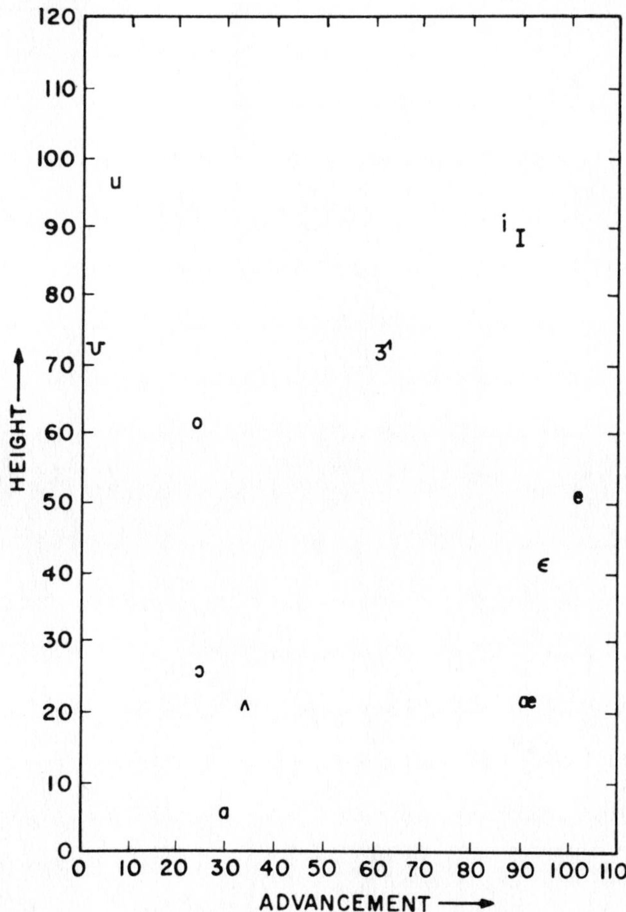

Figure 6-2. Plotting of the first two of the four-dimensional MDS output involving English vowel perception in word context. (From Singh and Woods, 1972; reprinted by permission.)

preted on dimension 1 and height on dimension 2. Figure 6-3 shows the plotting of dimensions 3 and 4. On the third dimension, the feature retroflexion seems to have been utilized (/ɝ/ is placed apart from all other vowels), and on the fourth dimension the feature lax/tense was retrieved. (Lax vowels /ʌ, ɛ, ʊ, ɪ, ɝ/ placed themselves separately from nonlax vowels /o, i, ɔ, ɑ, æ, u/.) It seems that the feature tenseness was retrieved when the vowels were presented in the context of meaningful words and was not retrieved when the vowels were presented in isolation (Singh and Woods, 1972). This result can be

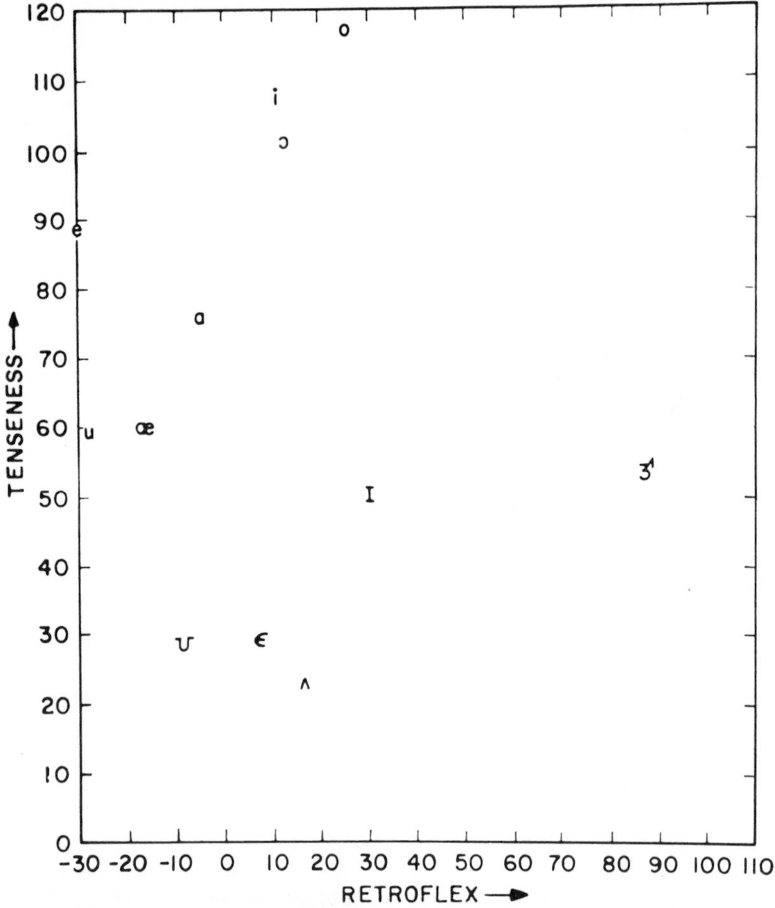

Figure 6-3. Plotting of dimensions 3 and 4 of the four-dimensional MDS output involving English vowel perception in word context. (From Singh and Woods, 1972; reprinted by permission.)

expected because the nontense vowels cannot occur in isolation in English and hence may not be perceived in isolation.

TERBEEK AND HARSHMAN (1971)

Terbeek and Harshman (1971) studied vowel perception cross-linguistically. The languages involved were German, English, and Thai. They found a two-dimensional solution, which was interpreted as tongue height and advancement for the English and Thai judges. A three-dimensional solution, height, advancement, and rounding, was found for the German subjects.

SHEPARD (1972)

Shepard (1972) reanalyzed the Peterson and Barney vowel confusion matrix involving 10 English vowels in meaningful words and recovered a three-dimensional vowel diagram with the perceptual attributes of advancement, height, and tenseness. Shepard correlated the F_1, F_2, and F_3 of the Peterson and Barney (1952) data to the rotated axes of the three perceptual dimensions and obtained high correlations. The rotation of the formant values against the perceptual coordinates showed a perceptually independent (orthogonal) nature of the first formant (approximately 90 degrees). However, a smaller angle between the higher formants (49 degrees) indicated their lack of independence in speech perception.

GRANT (1971)

Grant (1971) used eight vowels common to English and Hindi languages in the contexts of meaningful words in both of these languages. The consonantal contexts /b*V*t/ in English and /b*V*t̪/ in Hindi formed meaningful words for the vowels /i, ɪ, ɛ, ɑ, o, ʌ, ʊ, u/ in both of these languages. The stimuli were lowpass filtered at 9.5 kHz, sampled with 9-bit resolution at a rate of 18 kHz, and stored on a magnetic tape by a PDP-12 digital computer. The final /t/ for English speakers and /t̪/ for Hindi speakers were electronically truncated (to eliminate semantic variables), producing a uniform /b*V*/ segment for the Hindi and English vowels. The initial /b/ was retained in the stimuli in an attempt to add to the probability that the consonant-vowel syllable is perceived in the speech mode. Six native speakers of English and six native speakers of Hindi rated the dissimilarity of the stimuli of both languages on an eight-point equal appearing interval scale. The data were analyzed for each language separately and also in a combined condition.

The results of the two language groups were very consistent with each other. A final analysis in which both the listeners and speakers of Hindi and English were pooled and the vowels of the two languages were kept apart is shown in Figure 6-4 in a two-dimensional

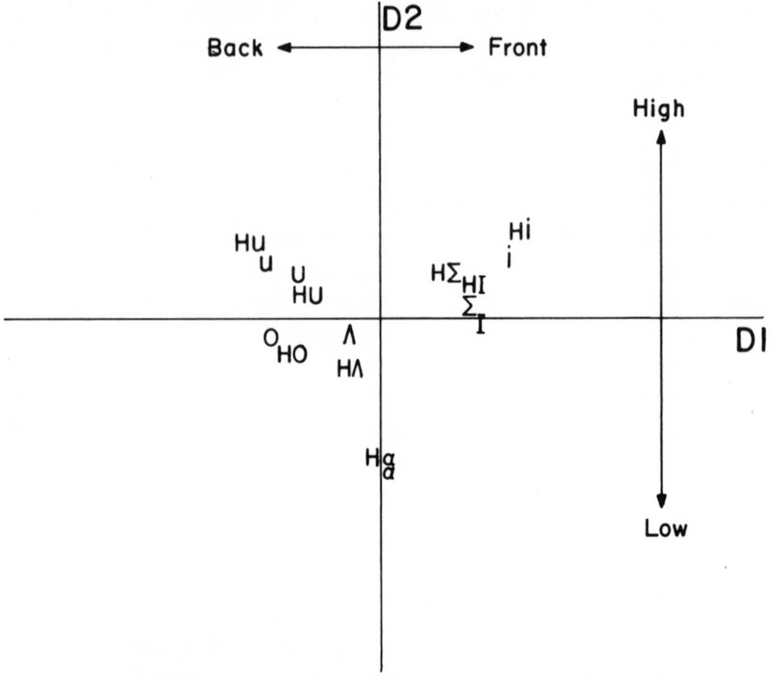

Figure 6-4. Plotting of INDSCAL dimensions 1 and 2 with the interpretations of advancement and height, respectively. Each vowel is represented twice, once for Hindi and once for English. (From Grant, 1971.)

space. The vowels just adjacent to H, in this figure, belong to the Hindi language, and the remaining vowels belong to the English language. This figure shows that: 1) Hindi and English vowels are extremely close to each other in a two-dimensional perceptual space, and 2) the eight vowels emerged in the traditional vowel diagram locations.

ROLE OF DISTINCTIVE FEATURES IN ARTICULATION AND SPEECH DISCRIMINATION

chapter 7
Distinctive Features and Language Acquisition

CONTENTS

Wellman et al. (1931)
Poole (1934)
Templin (1957)
Irwin (1947)
Nakazima (1962)
Snow (1963)
Bricker (1967)
Messer (1967)
Menyuk (1968)
Menyuk and Anderson (1969)
Cairns and Williams (1972)
Singh, Faircloth, and Faircloth (in press)
Singh's analysis of R. Irwin's data
Prather, Hedrick, and Kern (1975)
Markedness
Acquisition of phonetic features in children two to six years old—Frederick F. Weiner and John Bernthal (University of Maryland)

When children progress from the babbling stage of language development to the word stage in the hierarchy of phonological acquisition, they begin to learn the contrasts of phonemes that contribute to differences in meaning. The phonological contrasts are learned by contrasting components called distinctive features. The "words" /bɑ/ and /mɑ/ may be contrasted by very young children to signify two different objects, one of which may mean father and the other may mean mother. Each such contrast has an associated feature with specific commonality and differences. The child who differentiates /bɑ/ from /mɑ/ is contrasting the feature oral/nasal at the labial place of articulation. (The phonemes /b/ and /m/ share all features except oral/nasal.) The focal point of this chapter is to investigate how

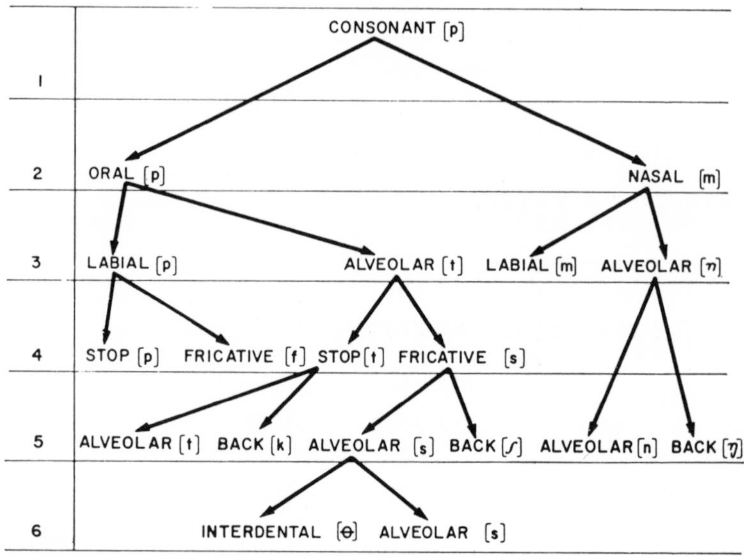

Figure 7-1. The developmental sequence of distinctive features. (From Singh and Frank, 1972.)

distinctive features can explain children's learning of phonemic contrasts.

Jakobson's hypothesis provides the background for describing some recent work in the area of phonological acquisition. Jakobson (1941, reprinted 1968) proposed that phonological acquisition is governed by the binary contrast of phonemes starting with the general differentiation of major phonetic classes and terminating at the phonemic level of adult phonology. Figure 7-1 shows the developmental sequence of distinctive features based on the Jakobson principle. There are six levels of feature development marked in this diagram. The first level indicates the phonemic contrast of the consonant /p/ and the vowel /ɑ/. The second level of acquisition shows the oral/nasal contrast, thus indicating the acquisition of the feature nasality (restricted to the labial place of articulation). The third level of the acquisition of distinctive features indicates the feature labiality, where the labial consonants /p/ and /m/ have been contrasted with the nonlabial (alveolar) consonants /t/ and /n/. The /p, m/ and /t, n/ are parallel pairs. The members of both of these pairs are similar by the same features and dissimilar by the same features. The fourth level of acquisition shows the distinction of /p/ and /f/ on the one hand and /t/

and /s/ on the other hand. This level indicates the acquisition of the feature continuancy. Thus far, i.e., up to the level 4, acquisition has involved the place of articulation of front sounds only. The fifth level shows acquisition of the front/back place contrast, thus indicating the acquisition of the distinction of /t/ from /k/, /s/ from /ʃ/, and /n/ from /ŋ/. The fourth and the fifth levels together signal the acquisition of the feature sibilancy. Finally, the sixth level shows the contrast of /θ/ with /s/, demonstrating that within the continuant category the −sibilant /θ/ is being distinguished from the +sibilant /s/.

The sequencing implicit in the Jakobson diagram indicates the following acquisition hierarchy: 1) nasality, 2) labiality, 3) continuancy, 4) front/back place, and 5) sibilancy. Because Jakobson is unclear regarding the acquisition of the voicing feature, simultaneous representation of the voiceless and voiced cognates has been provided here. Upon inspection of some developmental data, however, it will become clear that the +voice feature is generally acquired later than the −voiced feature.

WELLMAN ET AL. (1931)

The sequence of the acquisition of phonemes in the speech of young children has been determined by several investigators. Wellman et al. (1931) used 75% correct production of a sound as an arbitrary criterion for acquisition and reported data on the consonant phonemes of English. Table 7-1 shows the age, acquired phonemes, and the author's analysis of the acquisition of the distinctive features. Because of the criterion of 75% correct, these investigators were unable to

Table 7-1. Distinctive feature analysis of Wellman et al. (1931) data

Age (years)	Phoneme	Distinctive feature
3	/m, n, f, h, w, b/	Nasality, labiality, voicing, continuancy, sonorancy
4	/p, j, k, g, l/	Voicing
5	/d, r, s, tʃ, ʃ, v, t, z/	Front/back place, sibilancy
6	/dʒ/	

report the very early acquisition of the features of consonants. By age three, nasality, labiality, voicing, sonorancy, and continuancy have been acquired. Unless earlier data are reported for age nine months to three years, the sequence of these features cannot be determined.

It is difficult to determine feature acquisition from phonemic acquisition data not originally intended for feature analysis. A feature may have been acquired much earlier than shown in these data. Because the criterion for acquisition was 75% correct usage of a total phoneme, the correctly realized features were not counted as acquired. If a child made only a one-feature error, the remaining features of the phoneme were realized correctly, yet the entire phoneme was scored as incorrect. The use of the correct phoneme production criterion means that the acquisition of individual features cannot be accounted for. It is therefore important to recognize that the interpretation of feature development is extremely limited when only correct phonemic production is considered.

At age three, nasality is considered acquired because children distinguish /m, n/ from /f, h, w, b/. More specifically, nasality is the only feature that separates /m/ from /b/. The feature labiality is considered acquired because the labial consonants /m, w, b, f/ are distinguished from /n, h/, and more specifically, labiality is the only feature that distinguishes /m/ and /n/. The acquisition of the feature voicing may be inferred from the articulatory distinction of /f/ from the voiced phonemes. The acquisition of continuancy is evidenced by the distinctions of /f, h/ from the other consonants. The feature sonorancy distinguishes /w/ from /b/. At age four, voicing shows clear evidence of acquisition in the /k, g/ phoneme minimal pair. No other features are listed at age four on the table because they have been already acquired at age three. At age five, the features front/back place and sibilancy have been acquired. The phoneme pair /s/ and /ʃ/ share all features except front/back place. Although the back phonemes /k, g, h/ have been acquired earlier, the feature front/back place is not considered completely emerged until age five. At age three, the feature continuancy distinguishes /h/ from the other consonants.

At age four labiality can distinguish all acquired consonants. At age five mid and back place are acquired to allow the complete set of stops /p, t, k, b, d, g/ to emerge. At age five the feature sibilancy is also acquired to distinguish the phonemes /s, z, ʃ, tʃ/ from the nonsibilant phonemes.

An overall examination of these data indicates that the features nasality, labiality, sonorancy, voicing, and continuancy are acquired earlier than the features front/back place and sibilancy. It is interesting to compare the results of developmental feature acquisition strategies with the crossover points of features between the highpass and lowpass filters in Figure 5-4 plotted from the Miller and Nicely (1955) data. The features with crossover points at the lower end of the frequency spectrum are nasality, voicing, and frication, and the features with the crossover points at the higher end of the frequency spectrum are duration (sibilancy) and place of articulation. Thus, it may be concluded that the consonants with critical frequency elements at the lower end of the spectrum are acquired earlier than the consonants with critical frequency elements at the higher end of the spectrum.

POOLE (1934)

Poole (1934) reported phonemic acquisition when the criterion was set at 100% correct production. With this strict criterion for phonemic acquisition, the earliest age at which a phoneme could be considered acquired was 3.5 years. Starting to report acquisition at 3.5, Poole reported at every 12 months until the age of 7.5. Table 7-2 shows that the first five phonemes produced without error (at age 3.5) were /m, p, h, w, b/. These phonemes indicate the acquisition of nasality /m/, /b/, voicing /p/, /b/, labiality /m, p, w, b/, /h/, and sonorancy /b/, /w/. At age 4.5 front/back place was acquired, to include the phonemes /n, ŋ, j, k, d, g, t/ and to account for the distinctions of /p, t, k/, /b, d, g/, and /m, n, ŋ/. At age 5.5, the feature continuancy was acquired; continuancy

Table 7-2. Distinctive feature analysis of Poole (1934) data

Age (years)	Phoneme	Distinctive feature
3.5	/m, p, h, w, b/	Nasality, voicing, labiality, sonorancy
4.5	/n, ŋ, j, k, d, g, t/	Front/back place
5.5	/f/	Continuancy
6.5	/ʃ, v, l, ð, ʒ/	Sibilancy
7.5	/r, s, θ, z, ʍ/	

distinguishes /f/ from the already acquired /p/. Sibilancy is the last feature acquired, at age 6.5, when /ʃ, ʒ/ appear for the first time.

TEMPLIN (1957)

Table 7-3 shows the Templin (1957) data of acquisition of consonant phonemes at ages 3, 3.5, 4, 4.5, 6, and 7 years. The criterion for phonemic acquisition was also 75% correct. Table 7-3 shows that, although the acquisition of individual phonemes shows some differences, the overall ranking of feature acquisition is very much the same as above: the features nasality, sonorancy, labiality, voicing, and continuancy have been acquired before the features front/back place and sibilancy.

The Templin data also indicate the role that markedness plays in the acquisition of a consonant feature. The labial consonants have been acquired before all other consonants. The voiceless consonants of the voiceless/voiced cognates have been acquired before the voiced (exception /t/). Thus, /f/ is acquired before /v/; /p/ is acquired before /b/; /s/ is acquired before /z/; /ʃ/ is acquired before /ʒ/; /tʃ/ is acquired before /dʒ/; and /θ/ is acquired before /ð/. The phoneme pair /k, g/ has been acquired simultaneously. In addition, Table 7-3 also shows that the phonemes acquired latest contain the greatest number of marked features. The phonemes /ð, z, ʒ, dʒ, ʍ/ are marked for place, manner, and voicing.

Table 7-3. Distinctive feature analysis of Templin (1957) data

Age (years)	Phoneme	Distinctive feature
3	/m, n, ŋ, p, f, h, w/	Nasality, sonorancy, labiality, voicing, continuancy
3.5	/j/	
4	/k, b, d, g, r/	Front/back place
4–5	/s, ʃ, tʃ/	Sibilancy (voiceless)
6	/t, θ, v, l/	
7	/ð, z, ʒ, dʒ, ʍ/	Sibilancy (voiced)

The acquisition of phonemes reported by Wellman (1931), Poole (1934), and Templin (1957) all started at or beyond the three-year stage. However, it is well established that "most phonological learning occurs in the first three years of life" (Berko and Brown, 1960, p. 526). Therefore, in the preceding analyses we have been unable to develop a sequencing of distinctive feature acquisition. By age three, the children in these studies have already acquired most of the distinctive features with adequate proficiency.

IRWIN (1947)

Irwin (1947a,b) studied the acquisition of phonemes from infancy (age one to two months) to the age of 29 to 30 months. Figures 7-2 and 7-3 are reinterpretations of Irwin's profiles for consonant usage. These reinterpretations are based on manner, place, and voicing features. Figure 7-2 shows the acquisition of the phonetic features nasal, stop, continuant, and semivowels and glides. Other than the pooling of semivowels and glides, all other classifications are Irwin's. The

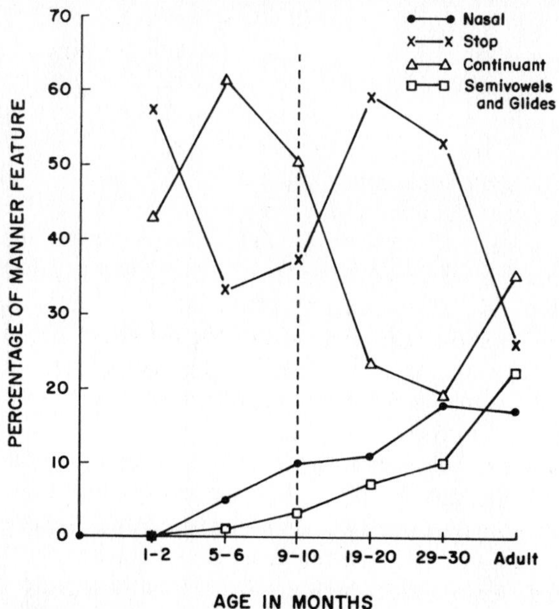

Figure 7-2. Acquisition of the features nasal, stop, continuant, and semivowel and glide as a function of age. (Based on Irwin, 1947.)

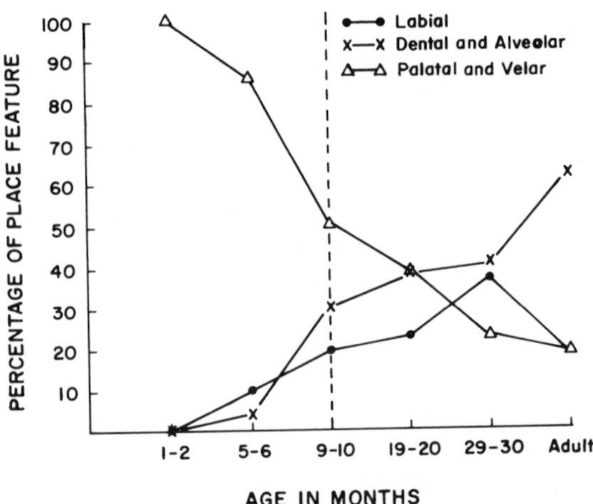

Figure 7-3. Acquisition of the features labial, dental and alveolar, and palatal and velar as a function of age. (Based on Irwin, 1947.)

abscissa in this figure shows the age, ranging from 1–2 months to 29–30 months, and the frequency of usage in adult speech (based on Voelker's (1945) count). The ordinate shows the percentage of manner features uttered. This figure shows that the phonetic features nasality and semivowels/glides emerge at five to six months and show steady growth. To the contrary, the phonetic features stop and continuant show erratic tendencies. Stops are used with greater frequency at the developmental stages than at the adult level. The stop curve, interpreted beyond the "first-word level" (nine to ten months) in the phonology of the average child, shows clearly that children during phonological development use an inordinately greater number of stops than any other category of sounds.

Figure 7-3 shows the trend of the acquisition of the three places of articulation (labial or front, dental and alveolar or mid, and palatal and velar or back). The abscissa, again, shows the age, ranging from 1–2 months to 29–30 months, with the frequency of adult usage. The ordinate shows the percentage of the place of articulation feature uttered. The palatal/velar place shows greater usage at the very early stages with almost a linearly descending trend until the curve reaches the adult stage. An opposite tendency may be observed for the dental/alveolar consonants, which are used less frequently at the very early stages with a steady increase in usage over time. Thus, at the 29- to 30-month stage, alveolar consonants are used most frequently, followed by labial consonants, and the velar/palatal consonants are used least frequently. The labial place of articulation is also used with greater frequency in the child's speech than in the adult's speech. Although both the labial and velar consonants are used with greater frequency in the child's speech, the difference between them is that the phonological usage of labials increases during the developmental stage but the usage of velars decreases.

Figure 7-4 shows the acquisition of the voiceless and voiced specifications of the voicing feature. The data used to draw these curves are based on only 14 of the voiceless/voiced cognates included in the Irwin studies. Thus, the nasals, semivowels, glides, glottal stops, and the fricative /h/ are not included in determining the frequency of usage of the voiceless and voiced categories. The curve representing voiceless consonants shows a steep rise over time while the voiced consonants show slow or no rate of increment.

An overall examination of the three curves representing the sequencing of phonetic features as a function of age reveals that the children's priority of features is very different from the adults' and that, with time, the children's system approximates more and more the system of adults. The crossing of several features between the early stages of development and the adult stage supports the above conclusion. As a matter of fact, it seems that the features used with greater frequency by young children are those used least by adults. The dichotomy in manner is obvious between stops and continuants, in place between velar and alveolar, and in voicing between voiced

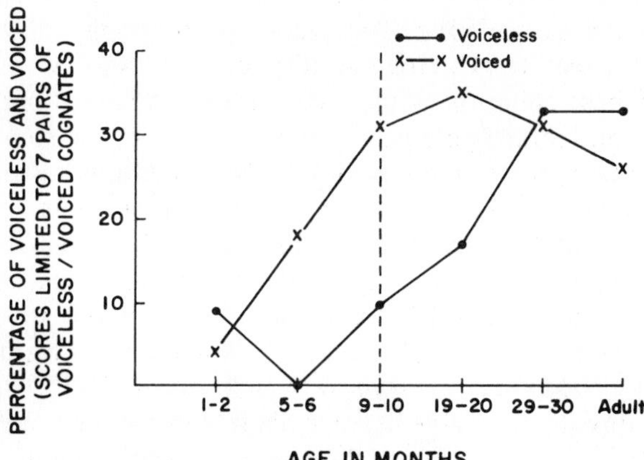

Figure 7-4. Acquisition of the features voiceless and voiced as a function of age. (Based on Irwin, 1947.)

and voiceless, manner being used more frequently by children and voicing by adults.

The phonetic feature analyses of the Wellman (1931), Poole (1934), Templin (1957), and Irwin (1947) data are all based on the transcription by these investigators. These transcriptions were mainly phonemic, or broad, based on the phonemic categories of the adult system. A narrow phonetic transcription of a very young child's speech would likely reveal an even more divergent system because the child's speech sounds would not be preclassified into the adult categories but rather examined in an unbiased manner.

NAKAZIMA (1962)

Nakazima (1962) studied six Japanese and four American children from birth to one year. Using acoustic and phonetic analyses, he described six developmental stages. The first two stages do not show any connection with articulatory development. The last four developmental stages—stages 3, 4, 5, and 6—reveal an important feature acquisition strategy. Front vowels are articulated along with a few labial consonants at *stage 3*. The age range associated with this stage is two to five months.

At *stage 4,* which has been called the stage of repetitive babbling, a more stable and elaborate representation of the labial consonants is present. The labial consonants dominating the speech production of these children were [b]-, [p]-, [w]-, [ɸ]-, and [v]-like sounds. In addition, some alveolar and palatal consonants, e.g., [d]-, [t]-, [dz]-, [tj]-, [ʎ]-like sounds, were also used. In a few cases the [k]-like sound, a velar stop, was also found. The sound spectrographic display indicated that the features voicing, nasality, and aspiration were utilized by most of these children. While the labiality component of the place of articulation feature emerged at the third stage, the fourth stage showed a much greater number of labials. In addition, alveolar and palatal contact also emerged at this stage, at about seven months.

At *stage 5* of development, an indication of the emergence of the features sibilancy and sonorancy could be deduced by the children's utilization of the [ʃ]- and [l]-like sounds. The children at this stage were nine months to one year old. The final developmental stage described by Nakazima was *stage 6,* which was marked by one-word utterances directly traceable to some adult words and phrases. These words show clear utilization of the features voicing, nasality, place, sonorancy, and continuancy. The children at this stage were all over one year old.

SNOW (1963)

Snow (1963) studied 438 first-grade children whose median age was seven years, two months. These children were given a picture vocabulary articulation test for consonants. The correct and error responses were tallied. Snow (1963) reported the confusion matrix for consonants as well as a reduced confusion matrix of the manner of articulation. As expected, these children acquired important phonetic features by this age. Except for the phonetic category of voiced fricative, all other manners of articulation were found correctly produced at least 95% of the time. The phonetic category voiced fricative was correctly produced 81% of the time. The voicing feature showed an interesting tendency. Although the voiced substitution for the voiceless consonant was only 1.2%, the voiceless substitution for the voiced consonant was 14%.

Utilizing the distinctive features labiality, front/back place, sonorancy, continuancy, sibilancy, and nasality, Singh further analyzed Snow's consonant confusion matrix, and found the following results. The greatest number of substitutions occurred for the feature continuancy (approximately 10%). All of these errors were unidirectional; i.e., continuants were replaced by stops but not vice versa. The second degree of feature error was for the front/back place (approximately 3.4%), in which there was a greater tendency for the front consonant to substitute the back rather than vice versa. The third degree of feature error occurred for the feature sibilancy (approximately 2%). Singh's reanalysis of the Snow (1963) data shows a smaller percentage of errors for the fricative (continuant) than originally reported by Snow because he analyzed strictly distinctive feature errors while Snow analyzed only the phonetic errors. For example, in the Singh analysis, although /z/ replaced /ʒ/ 9.5% of the time, it would not be counted as a fricative error because it itself was a fricative consonant. However, if one only examines what consonants were erred, disregarding what the substitution phoneme was, then this 9.5% would be added toward penalizing the children as having a fricative error. In a proper system of counting feature errors, this is not a fricative error because the substituting phoneme is also a fricative.

Singh subjected the errors reported in Snow's experiment to a multidimensional analysis (INDSCAL) to determine the nature of distinctive features that may account for the consonant production errors. Figure 7-5 shows the recovery of the features voicing and sibilancy in the confusions of 15 obstruent consonants.

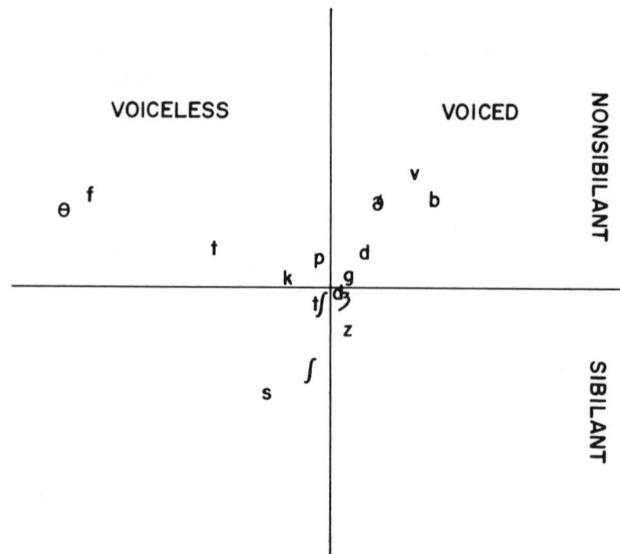

Figure 7-5. Plotting of dimensions 1 and 2 of a four-dimensional solution of Snow's data. (Reanalysis by Singh.)

BRICKER (1967)

Bricker (1967) analyzed the imitative behavior of 90 preschool children ages 3.0 to 3.9, 4.0 to 4.9, and 5.0 to 5.9 years by analyzing errors of place, manner, and voicing. Although Bricker claims that "the quantitative method for determining which of the components was preserved in the error responses was taken from Miller and Nicely (1955)," actually, the data reported in this study are limited to "mean percentage of specific, sound components" (p. 74). It may be recalled that Miller and Nicely determined the amount of information transmitted by each feature of their system.

In Bricker's report, the percentage of specific speech sound components of place, manner, and voicing is tallied for each of the three age groups. The voicing component shows maximal precision in elicited repetition (89% for 5.0 to 5.9 years; 88% for 4.0 to 4.9 years; and 76% for 3.0 to 3.9 years) and the place component the minimal precision (5% for 5.0 to 5.9 years; 8% for 4.0 to 4.9 years; and 18% for 3.0 to 3.9 years). The manner feature was considered of intermediate importance between voicing and place. The percentages pertaining to the place of articulation were pooled for bilabial, linguadental, postdental, palatal, and glottal[ʔ], while the manner of articulation was pooled for nasals, plosives, fricatives, and semivowels. The rationale for these specific classifications as well as the unexpected deterioration of the place of articulation with the increment in age was not explained. On the basis of the gross phonetic feature analysis (place, manner, and voicing), Bricker (1967) concluded his paper by claiming that: "the appropriate unit of behavior in the analysis of echoic responses is the component rather than the sounds as total units. A speech sound error response was generally controlled correctly by components along one or two of the three dimensions. These findings suggest that training focused on the place of articulation alone would be the most efficient way in which to bring the majority of echoic responses under appropriate stimulus control" (p. 75).

MESSER (1967)

Messer (1967) presented pairs of words to children three years, seven months old. These pairs were comprised of English and non-English words. The children were asked to judge which of the words in a pair sounded more like an English word. The children's judgments were analyzed by Jakobson, Fant, and Halle's (1952) distinctive feature system. The distinctive feature analysis of the substitution errors revealed that the large majority of the words were changed by one distinctive feature difference. It was concluded by Messer that when a child mispronounces a non-English word by substituting a phoneme, he is likely to make the changes minimal by moving the word into a category "very close to the original one, and by so doing, to make it more English" (p. 612).

MENYUK (1968)

The role of distinctive features in the acquisition of phonology of Japanese and American children was investigated by Menyuk (1968). The distinctive features gravity, diffuseness, stridency, nasality, continuancy, and voicing were used to analyze the phonological acquisition of children on the one hand and to predict the rank order of phonemic recall by the adult subjects on the other. In addition, the articulation performance of children was also rank ordered utilizing these features as criteria. The Japanese children were tested between the ages one and three years at eight different intervals. The American children were tested between the ages of two and five years at six different intervals.

Figures 7-6 and 7-7 show the plotting of the percentage of feature usage (ordinate) as a function of age (abscissa). Figure 7-6 shows the features used by the American children, and Figure 7-7 shows the features used by the Japanese children. The rank order of features in these languages was identical: 1) nasality, 2) gravity, 3) voicing, 4) diffuseness, 5) continuancy, and 6) stridency. Because syllables rather than words were the criterion for eliciting phonemic responses, the difference in the age factor was not considered crucial. It may be noted that the rank order of the feature acquisition in the Japanese and

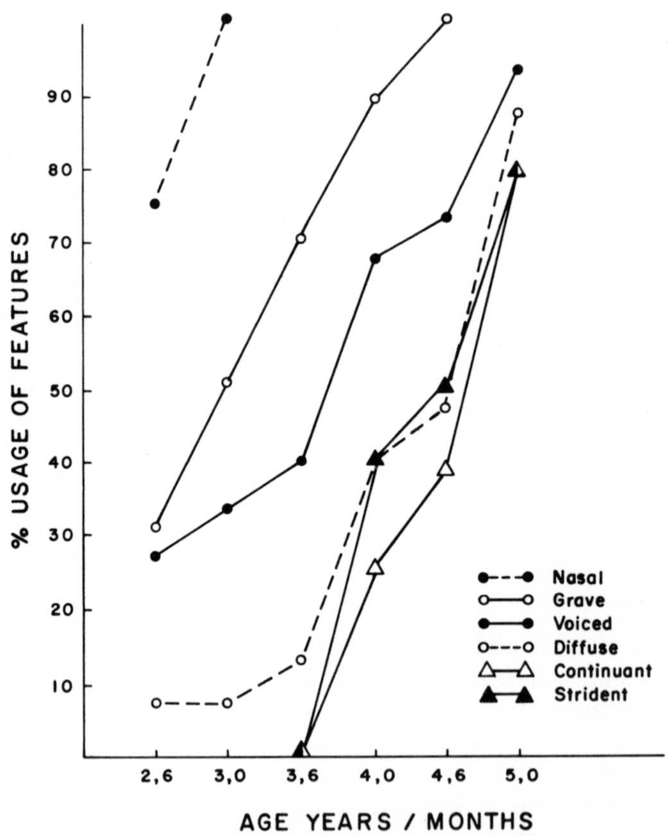

Figure 7-6. Acquisition of the features nasal, grave, voiced, diffuse, continuant, and strident as a function of age in American children. (From Menyuk, 1968; reprinted by permission.)

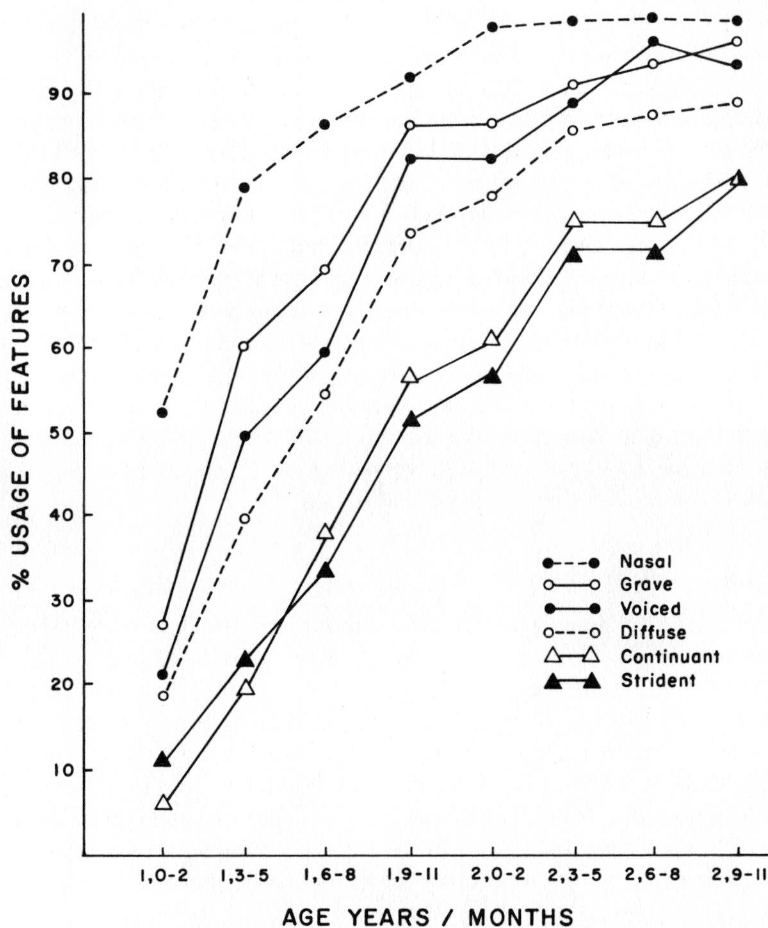

Figure 7-7. Acquisition of the features nasal, grave, voiced, diffuse, continuant, and strident as a function of age in Japanese children. (From Menyuk, 1968; reprinted by permission.)

American children was highly consistent with Jakobson's model described earlier.

MENYUK AND ANDERSON (1969)

Menyuk and Anderson (1969) examined the identification and reproduction of speech sounds /w/, /r/, and /l/ by preschool children. The stimuli for this experiment were synthetically prepared, involving the words *white*, *write*, and *light*. The results of this study showed that differences existed between the identification and reproduction tasks. A greater number of children responded correctly in the identification task than in the reproduction task. A significantly greater number of children produced the /w/ phoneme correctly as compared with the /l/ and /r/ phonemes. The fact that identification boundaries were correct a greater number of times than the reproduction boundaries led these authors to hypothesize that: "the developmental sequence in the acquisition of the members of this speech sound set is, first, the ability to identify differences between the members of the set and, second, the ability to reproduce the differences" (p. 40). The fact that a significantly greater number of /w/ responses was produced correctly was attributed to the +gravity nature of /w/ as compared with the −gravity nature of /l/ and /r/. It may be recalled that Jakobson's (1968) proposal identified labials, which are specified as +grave sounds, as the earliest learned feature.

CAIRNS AND WILLIAMS (1972)

Cairns and Williams examined the articulation errors of 384 children drawn equally from grades 1 to 12. The data were analyzed for substitution, omission, and distortion errors of 22 English consonants. The portion of results of interest here is the application of phonetic features (Chomsky and Halle, 1968) to the analysis of the substitution process. First, Cairns and Williams examined the substitution errors in light of the major class feature. They concluded that: "substitutes and targets are always of the same class of sounds. Thus, a glide never substitutes for an obstruent or vice versa" (p. 817).

The results pertaining to the place of articulation features revealed that maximal errors occurred for the coronal feature. However, all errors within this feature showed directionality of +coronal to −coronal and never a change of −coronal to +coronal. Thus, there were /f/ substituting for /θ/, and /w/ substituting for /l/, but not vice versa. The error pattern for the anterior feature showed the tendency of +anterior substituting for −anterior targets. Thus, /s/ was generally the substitute for /ʃ/, /t/ for /tʃ/, and /d/ for /dʒ/.

The direction of the place feature errors can be explained by the ease of production. For manner of articulation, there was an overwhelming tendency for the continuancy feature to be in error, with 65 out of 70 errors showing a unidirectional tendency. The +continuant target was replaced by −continuant sounds (also see Singh and Frank, 1972). The voicing feature also showed unidirectional error tendencies. In 48 out of 61 voicing errors, the +voice target was replaced by −voice. Cairns and Williams concluded that: "when the substitutions themselves are analyzed within a phonetic feature framework, it appears that individual substitutions can be explained by considerations of ease of articulation and perceptual distinctiveness" (pp. 818–819).

SINGH, FAIRCLOTH, AND FAIRCLOTH (IN PRESS)

Singh, Faircloth, and Faircloth (in press) analyzed tape-recorded samples of spontaneous connected conversational speech samples, approximately 60 seconds long, of 25 trainable mentally retarded youngsters. A series of scores was obtained on each of the 25 subjects for the phonetic categories of place, manner, and voicing for consonants, and mandibular movement and tongue-arch position for vowels. Scores were also obtained on the correct usage of syllables, morphemes, lexical classes, and function-word classes. In addition, the speech samples were judged for percentage of rated intelligibility.

A series of multiple correlations was obtained between the phonetic features of vowels and consonants and the rated intelligibility, syllabic integrity (unity of a syllable form), lexical classes, and function-word classes. The phonetic features of manner, place, and voicing correlated significantly at the 0.01 level of confidence with the rated intelligibility. The individual correlation was highest between the place of articulation and rated intelligibility, with the next correlation value being equal for both manner and voicing. The phonetic features of manner, place, and voicing also correlated significantly at the 0.01 level with the integrity of the various types of syllables. The individual correlation was the highest between voicing and syllabic integrity. This correlation was 0.89, which was as high as the multiple correlation value itself. Therefore, not much interpretive value was assigned to the high correlation of manner and place features with the integrity of syllable types. The distinctive phonetic features of vowels also correlated with the rated intelligibility significantly at the 0.01 level.

Although the intelligibility rating of the conversational speech was predicted by the distinctive phonetic features of consonants and vowels, it was not predicted significantly by the lexical and function-word classes. Thus, it was concluded that the phonetic features of consonants and vowels may be considered governed by the surface level grammar (phonetic rules) whereas the morphemic, lexical, and function-word classes may be governed by the deep level grammar (higher level rules).

Mean percentage scores were obtained for eight phonetic categories of place of articulation, five phonetic categories of manner of articulation, and two phonetic categories of voicing. The ordering revealed that bilabial place was most frequently produced correctly and that the linguadental place was least frequently produced correctly. Alveolar place was third to last in the frequency of correct production. This represents a serious deterrent to the articulatory proficiency of this group because many English consonants are alveolar. Furthermore, three (/s, t, n/) of the five most commonly used consonants are alveolar. While the fricative manner of production in general was very poorly produced, a specification of correct productions in different places of articulation was more variable. Glottal and labiodental fricatives held high ranks whereas linguadental and linguaalveolar fricatives held low ranks. The specification of the voicing categories indicated that voiceless consonants held higher rank than the voiced consonants (Singh and Frank, 1972).

An examination of the standard deviations associated with the mean percentage of correct scores indicated little variability among the 25 subjects for nasality and bilabial place; median variability for fricatives, stops, voicing, glides, and velar place; and greater variability for linguadental, glottal, labiodental, palatal place, and affricate. It is interesting to note that the features learned earlier were less variable and more stable than features learned later.

SINGH'S ANALYSIS OF R. IRWIN'S DATA

Irwin used 40 children in five age groups—ranging from four years, eleven months to eight years, one month—for collecting normative data in the domains of speech production and speech perception. These children responded to phonemes in the context of meaningful words, nonsense syllables, and prompting phrases. The errors were tallied for each of these contexts at the prevocalic and postvocalic word positions. In spite of the contextual constraints, the seven- and eight-year-old children made very few errors. Some errors in the production of consonants were seen for the five- and six-year-old children.

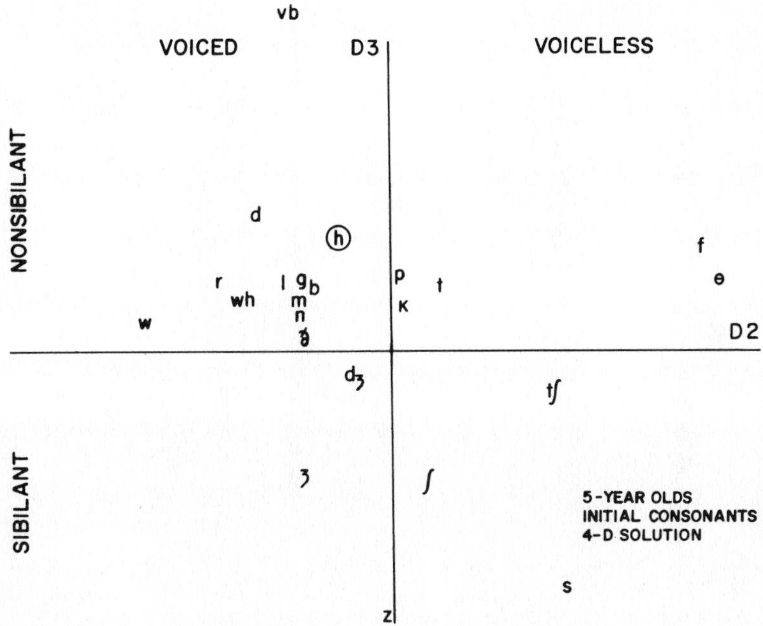

Figure 7-8. Plotting of dimensions 2 and 3 of a four-dimensional solution of the consonant confusions at the initial position. The speakers were five-year-old children.

Singh* performed INDSCAL analysis on the errors made by the five- and six-year-old children to investigate the role of distinctive features. Some examples of the results of the INDSCAL analysis are presented in Figure 7-8 for the five-year-old children and in Figure 7-9 for the six-year-old children. Figure 7-8 shows the production features of the five-year-old children when the consonant errors were made at the initial position of a word or a syllable. Two of the four dimensions are plotted in this figure. Dimension 2 has been interpreted as the voicing feature, which has separated all the voiceless consonants from the voiced ones. Dimension 3 has been interpreted as the sibilancy dimension, which separates the sibilant consonants /s, z, ʃ, tʃ, ʒ, dʒ/ from the nonsibilant consonants. The features utilized by the five-year-old children at the word-final position were voicing, continuancy, lip rounding, and linguadental place.

---

*Gratitude is expressed to Dr. Ruth B. Irwin of the Ohio State University who loaned this author the raw data for the INDSCAL analysis.

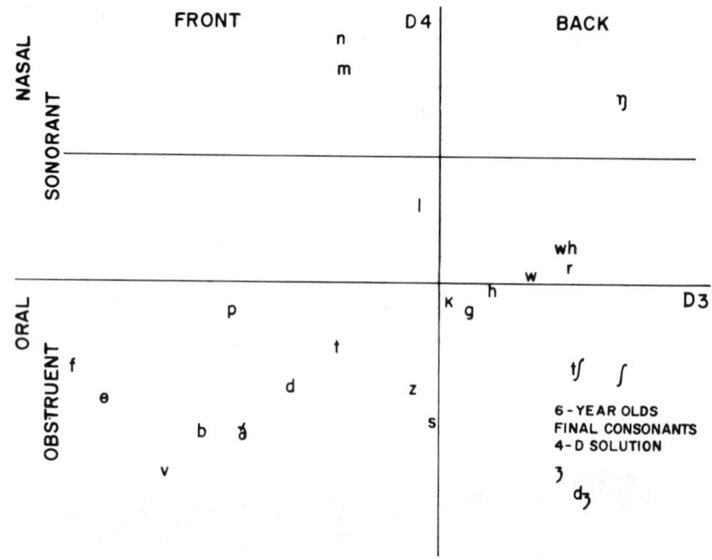

Figure 7-9. Plotting of dimensions 3 and 4 of a four-dimensional solution of the consonant confusions at the final position. The speakers were six-year-old children.

Some examples of the retrieval of the production features of the six-year-old children are shown in Figure 7-9. Dimension 3 shows the major class separation of obstruent consonants from the sonorant consonants. The sonorants are further divided into the nasal and the oral consonants. Dimension 4 separates the front from the back consonants.

The production features retrieved from the errors of the five-year-old and six-year-old children both at the prevocalic and post-vocalic positions in the INDSCAL analysis revealed the utilization of the features lip rounding, continuancy, voicing, sibilancy, labiality, sonorancy, and nasality. None of these features was retrieved at either position (initial or final) or age group. The retrieval by INDSCAL analysis of features in these conditions depends on the incidences of errors. Because these children did not make enough errors in all consonant categories, some of the features could not be retrieved consistently.

PRATHER, HEDRICK, AND KERN (1975)

The articulation development in 147 children ranging in age from 24 to 48 months was traced in terms of the distinctive features of consonants. Included in this study were 21 children each of the ages of 24, 28, 32, 36, 40, 44, and 48 months. Children exhibiting developmental problems or hearing difficulties were eliminated from the study. The responses were elicited by a photoarticulation test. The results were analyzed by the features nasality, voicing, gravity, diffuseness, continuancy, and stridency. These are the same features that Menyuk (1968) used to report the distinctive feature development of the English and Japanese children. Prather, Hedrick, and Kern (1975) plotted the correct production of distinctive features (in the error responses of these children) as a function of age. Figure 7-10 shows the plotting of the correct production of the plus specification of the nasality, voicing, gravity, diffuseness, continuancy, and stridency features. The abscissa in this figure shows age in months and the ordinate shows the percentage of correct feature production.

This figure compares the results obtained in the Prather, Hedrick, and Kern experiment (solid lines) with those of Menyuk's (1968) study (dotted lines) reported earlier. Although the trends of the two sets of curves in both studies are similar, it is evident from these figures that features appeared earlier in the children investigated by Prather, Hedrick, and Kern than the children investigated by Menyuk. The rank order of the features in terms of the maximal level of performance reached was: 1) nasal, 2) grave, 3) diffuse, 4) voiced, 5) continuant, and 6) strident, in the Prather, Hedrick, and Kern experiment; and 1) nasal, 2) grave, 3) voiced, 4) diffuse, 5) strident, and 6) continuant, in the Menyuk study.

Prather, Hedrick, and Kern also presented a comparison of the development of the plus and minus specifications of the six features. The plotting of these results is shown in Figure 7-11. Again, the abscissa in this figure represents age in months and the ordinate represents the percentage of correctly produced features. The solid line indicates the plus specification of a feature and the dotted line indicates the minus specification. The rank order of acquisition of the minus specifications of the features was not consistent with the rank order of the plus specifications.

MARKEDNESS

Figure 7-11 also can be examined from the markedness point of view. It is clear in the two bottom graphs that the minus specifications of the continuancy and stridency features consistently showed better articulation performance than the plus specification. It is generally believed

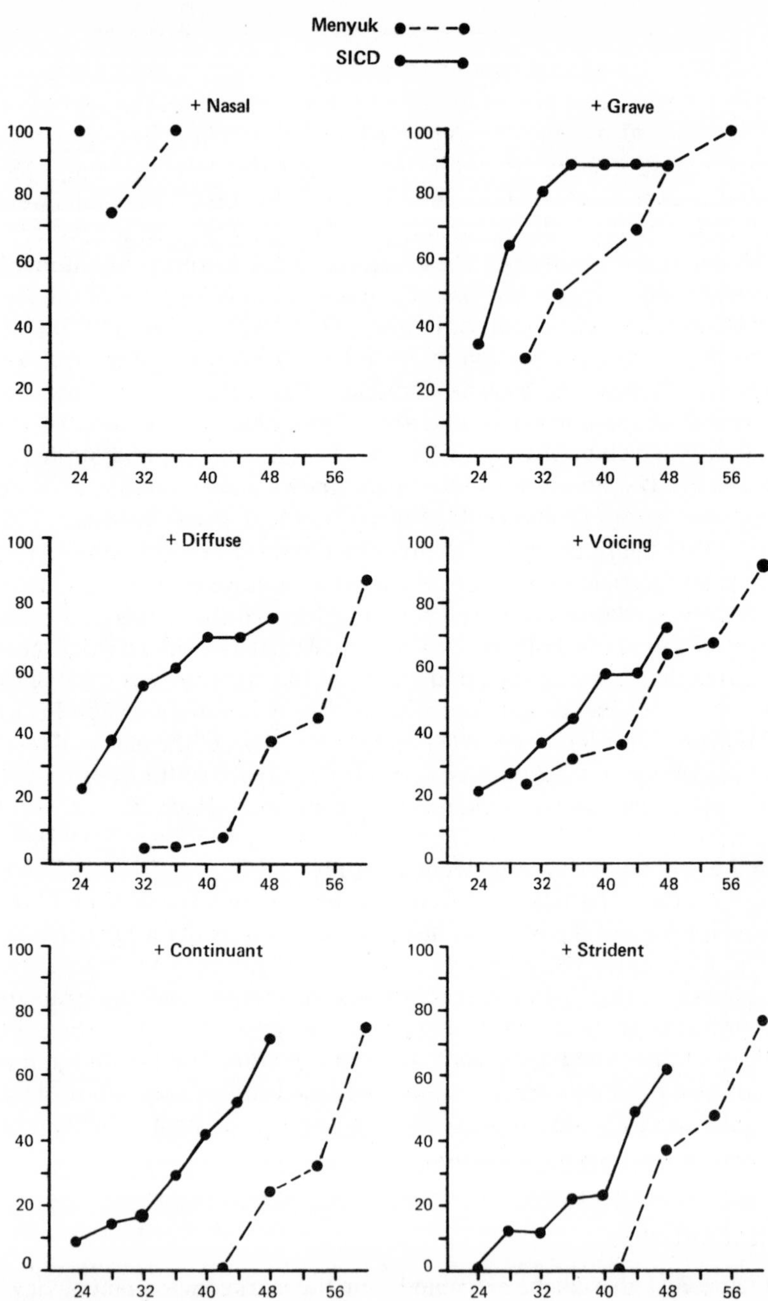

Figure 7-10. Comparison of Menyuk (1968, p. 140) and SICD analyses of correct plus feature usage for children 24 to 60 months of age. The vertical axis represents the percentage of correct productions of consonant sounds grouped according to the distinctive feature system of Jacobsen et al. (1963). The horizontal axis represents age in months. (From Prather, Hedrick, and Kern, 1975.)

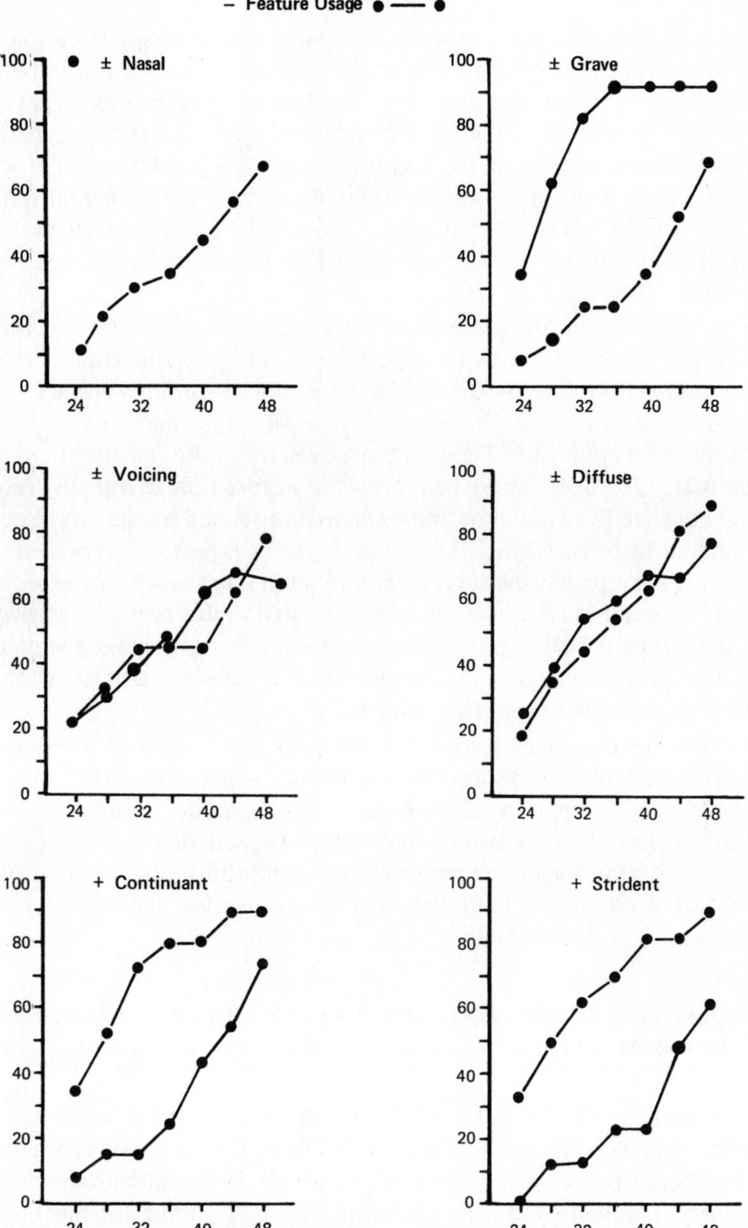

Figure 7-11. SICD data showing plus/minus feature contrasts for children 24 to 48 months of age. The vertical axis represents the percentage of correct productions of consonant sounds grouped according to the distinctive feature system of Jacobsen et al. (1963). The horizontal axis represents age in months. (From Prather, Hedrick, and Kern, 1975.)

that +continuant and +strident are marked feature specifications. Presence of markedness implies greater articulatory complexities and hence poor developmental index. The feature specification −grave (which is essentially −labial) is considered marked. Because of the presence of markedness, the −grave feature has greater articulatory complexities than the +grave (labial) feature. Developmental data shown in the upper right graph of Figure 7-11 show much better performance for the +grave (unmarked) feature than for the −grave (marked) feature.

Two kinds of literature have been discussed so far, studies that were not designed for distinctive feature analysis and studies that were. The first type is discussed here mainly for the purpose of providing background. For example, the phonemic substitution data of Wellman, Poole, and Templin have been interpreted with the aid of distinctive features. These reinterpretations are only marginally reliable because they are superimposed on the responses that were not meant for feature analysis. The second type of experiment reported in this chapter is purely distinctive feature analysis of children's speech. Menyuk's and Messer's studies are included in this type. An overall examination of both types of studies essentially reveals very similar findings regarding the utilization of distinctive features in the phonemic acquisition of the children.

The developmental studies reported so far in this chapter deal with distinctive features via the concept of the phoneme. The following study by Weiner and Bernthal is a significant departure from the other works in that the authors have directly used distinctive features as the criterion for phonemic development, without the intervening concept of phoneme. They have been kind to allow the inclusion of their study in this chapter.

ACQUISITION OF PHONETIC FEATURES IN CHILDREN TWO TO SIX YEARS OLD/*Frederick F. Weiner and John Bernthal (University of Maryland)*

Investigations of the order of feature acquisition have used three basic analysis techniques. They are: 1) phonological analysis of children's speech (Leopold, 1947; Weir, 1962); 2) identification of the features maintained during children's speech sound substitutions (Menyuk, 1968); and 3) calculations of the occurrence of specific features in speech sounds used correctly (Menyuk, 1968). Based on results from these investigations, inferences were made about the acquisition of feature contrasts using phonemic features. Hence, theoretical systems were used to generalize about nontheoretical (phonetic) events. This investigation was designed to demonstrate a methodology for evaluating feature acquisition with a phonetic feature system and to provide normative information relative to the feature errors that occurred in selected consonants produced by normally developing children.

Phonetic Feature System

The feature system utilized in this investigation was a modification of the phonetic feature system of Chomsky and Halle (1968). The phonetic features included for investigation represent articulatory movements inherent in the production of English phones. These articulatory maneuvers were assumed to be critical for the correct articulation of sounds in which they occurred.

The phonetic feature system referred to above is presented in Table 7-4. In view of phonetic and phonological theory, a few *apologia* are required. First, this feature system represents what the speaker takes to be certain phonetic properties of an utterance. Because the features are strictly articulatory descriptions, the phonetic properties are only partially related to the speaker's phonological rules. Second, this feature system was not intended to represent the phonetic capabilities of man or to provide an exhaustive list of features necessary to completely describe English phones. Third, the feature system was language specific and not intended to have universal application. Rather, it was designed to aid in the investigation of the acquisition of articulatory movements which occur during the production of selected English consonants.

Subjects

Subjects were 250 children enrolled in private preschools, nursery schools, or day-care centers in the Maryland suburbs of Washington, D.C., near College Park, Maryland. The sample consisted of 50 two-year-old children with a mean age of two years, seven months and ranging in age from two years to two years, eleven months (23 males and 27 females); 67 three-year-olds with a mean age of three years, six months and ranging in age from three years, one month to three years, 11 months (30 males and 37 females); 69 four-year-olds with a mean age of four years, seven months and ranging in age from four years, two months to four years, eleven months (34 males and 35 females); and 59 five-year-olds with a mean age of five years, five

Table 7-4. Brief articulatory descriptions of the positive characters of each phonetic feature used in this investigation

Feature[a]	Articulatory description
Anterior	Made with primary constriction forward of the alveo-palatal region
Coronal	Made with the blade of the tongue
High	Made with the tongue body raised from the neutral position
Back	Made with the tongue body retracted and slightly raised from the neutral position
Low	Made with the tongue body lowered from the neutral position
Distributed	Made with a relatively long constriction in the oral cavity
Nasal	Made with an abnormally large velopharyngeal valve opening
Lateral	Made with a side channel for air flow created by lowering one or both sides of the tongue
Delayed Release	Made by creating a narrow passageway so turbulence can be generated during the brief period immediately following release of the articulators
Continuant	Produced with the primary constriction in the vocal tract, not narrowed enough to completely constrict the air flow
Voice	Produced with vocal fold vibration

[a]All features describe consonants.

months and ranging in age from five years to five years, eleven months (26 males and 33 females). All children were white and were assumed to be from middle-class socioeconomic homes. Subjects had no known intellectual, learning, neurological, or physiological handicapping conditions according to school records and teacher judgments.

Examiners

Ten upper-level undergraduate students were trained to evaluate articulation in young children using the above feature system. Each examiner, as part of his academic preparation, had completed at least one course in phonetics and one in articulation disorders before being trained as an examiner. Examiners participated in a 12-hour training program. After the program, trainees took a skills test that required evaluation of 22 sound productions. A criterion of 95% agreement with the senior author was required in judging 121 features within 23 phonemes. In addition, each feature complex of 11 features per phone had to be scored in 10 seconds or less. Trainees unable to meet these criteria received additional training until they met criteria or were dropped from the program.

Stimuli

The stimuli consisted of 84 pictures used to elicit productions of 23 consonants. Each sound was represented twice in the prevocalic position and twice in the postvocalic position with the exception of /ʒ/ and /ŋ/, which were only represented in the postvocalic position, and /w/ and /j/, which were only represented in the prevocalic position.

Elicitation Procedure

Each examiner tested 25 children between two and six years of age. Responses were evaluated during the production of each target sound and were elicited using picture stimuli. When a stimulus item did not evoke the appropriate picture label, the child was instructed to imitate the examiner's production. After the presentation of two more stimulus items, the original inappropriately named picture stimulus was again presented and this production was scored. In the event that a child still did not label the picture appropriately, an imitative response was scored. Imitative responses comprised a small proportion of the total number of responses obtained.

Scoring

Each target phoneme was evaluated with the aid of a template. Each template included a listing of the idealized features for each phoneme. In actual practice these templates served as a list of "yes/no" questions, one question for each of the 11 feature contrasts in the system. The checklist of questions corresponding to the /f/ template is presented in Table 7-5. Each "no" answer to these questions was scored

Table 7-5. Checklist of questions corresponding to the /f/ template

1. Was the target produced with primary constriction forward of the alveolar ridge?
2. Was the target produced without the blade of the tongue?
3. Was the target produced without raising the tongue body from the neutral position?
4. Was the target produced without lowering the tongue body from the neutral position?
5. Was the target produced without a retracted tongue body?
6. Was the target produced with a relatively short constriction in the oral cavity?
7. Was the target produced with the velopharyngeal valve in the closed mode?
8. Was the target produced without a side channel for air flow?
9. Was the target produced so that when the articulators were released there was not a brief period when a narrow passageway was formed and turbulence generated in the vocal tract?
10. Was the target produced so that the primary constriction did not completely obstruct the air flow?
11. Was the target produced without vocal fold vibration?

as an error. For example, an answer of "no" to the first question (Was the sound produced anterior to the hard palate?) would indicate that the child's attempt to produce /f/ resulted in a production whose primary constriction was posterior to the alveolar ridge. A "no" answer to the second question (Was the sound produced without the blade of the tongue?) would indicate that the child's attempt to produce /f/ resulted in a production in which the blade of the tongue was involved. This procedure was followed until the corresponding question for each of the 11 features was answered.

This methodology represents a departure from the procedures where the features of substituted phonemes are compared to the features of target phonemes and differences are scored as errors (Menyuk, 1968). The major advantage of the present system is that it allows for the evaluation of all articulation errors whether they be substitutions, omissions, or distortions.

Results and Discussion

The proportion of errors on each specific feature was computed separately for fricatives, sonorants, and stops in the pre- and postvocalic positions. The proportion of feature errors in affricates and stops was pooled and referred to as stops in all figures and discussion. Subjects in this investigation made relatively few errors during production of the following phonetic features: −low (+low does not occur for consonants), +nasal, −lateral, and −voice. The proportion of errors at each level for the plus and minus characters of each feature is presented, with the exception of −low, in Figures 7-12 to 7-31. Data from −low were excluded because the proportion of errors was always zero for this feature.

Anterior The proportion of errors on +anterior during the production of fricatives /f/, /v/, /θ/, /ð/, /s/, and /z/; sonorants /l/, /m/, and /n/; stops /p/, /b/, /t/, and /d/ for each age level can be seen in Figure 7-12. The percentage of errors plotted in Figure 7-12 represents the proportion of times that subjects produced sounds posterior to the alveolar ridge when the idealized phoneme target had a place of articulation in the oral cavity anterior to the alveolar ridge. It can be seen that, except in the case of prevocalic sonorants, subjects made 5% errors or less on +anterior at two years of age. Errors on +anterior in prevocalic sonorants were 7% by two years of age and only 3% at three years of age.

The proportion of errors on −anterior for pre- and postvocalic stops /k/, /g/, /tʃ/, and /dʒ/; fricatives /ʃ/ and /ʒ/; and sonorants /w/, /r/, /j/, and /ŋ/ for each age level is presented in Figure 7-13. The sonorant /ŋ/ was presented only in the postvocalic position, and /w/ and /j/ only in the prevocalic position. Errors on −anterior represented productions at or anterior to the alveolar ridge when the idealized production was posterior to the alveolar ridge. When Figures 7-12 and 7-13 are compared, it can be seen that a much higher proportion of errors occurred on −anterior than on +anterior. At the earliest age tested (two to three years), −anterior was in error more than 5% in all classes of sounds. By three years of age −anterior errors were significantly reduced, and by four years of age errors were almost nonexistent, with the exception of those within postvocalic fricatives.

There were more errors for the anterior feature during the production of /ʃ/, /ʒ/, /tʃ/, /dʒ/, /k/, and /g/ (the −anterior stops and

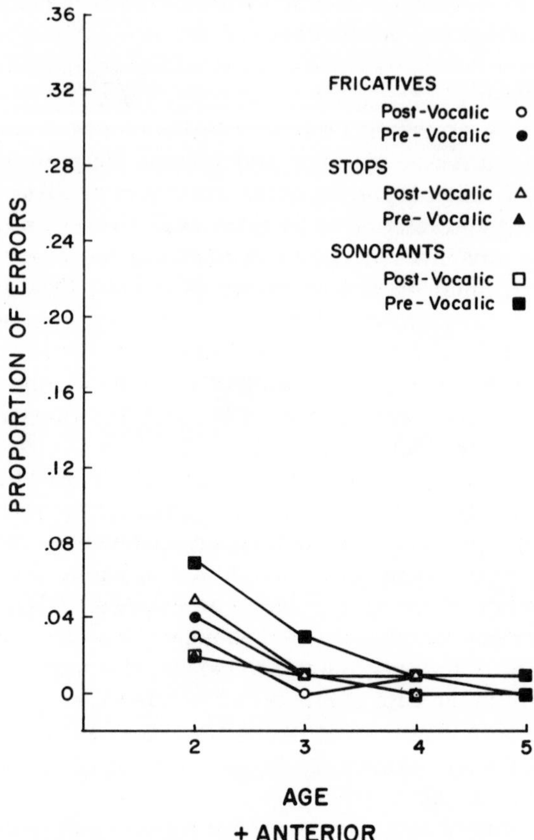

Figure 7-12. The proportion of +anterior errors for pre- and postvocalic fricatives, stops, and sonorants in children two to six years of age.

fricatives) than for all other sounds examined. This result would be predicted from markedness theory (Chomsky and Halle, 1968; Cairns, 1969) because these sounds are the only ones marked for anterior (Cairns and Cairns, 1971).

Coronal The proportion of errors for +coronal during the production of pre- and postvocalic fricatives /θ/, /ð/, /s/, /z/, /ʃ/, and /ʒ/; sonorants /l/, /r/, and /n/; and stops /t/, /d/, /tʃ/, and /dʒ/ at each age level is presented in Figure 7-14. Errors on +coronal were instances where a sound should have been but was not produced with the corona or front portion of the tongue.

It can be seen from the results in Figure 7-14 that +coronal was in error 10 to 18% at two years of age in fricatives and sonorants, but only 1 to 4% in stops. At five years +coronal had dropped to 1 to 3% errors in sonorants but remained at 7 to 8% in fricatives. An obvious developmental trend is seen in the reduction of coronal errors within sonorants and fricatives. Plus coronal in stops never exceeded an error rate of 4%, even in the two-year-old group.

The higher proportion of +coronal errors in fricatives and sonorants would be predicted from Menyuk's (1972) hypothesis. Menyuk (1972) states that sounds which are mastered late involve "manipula-

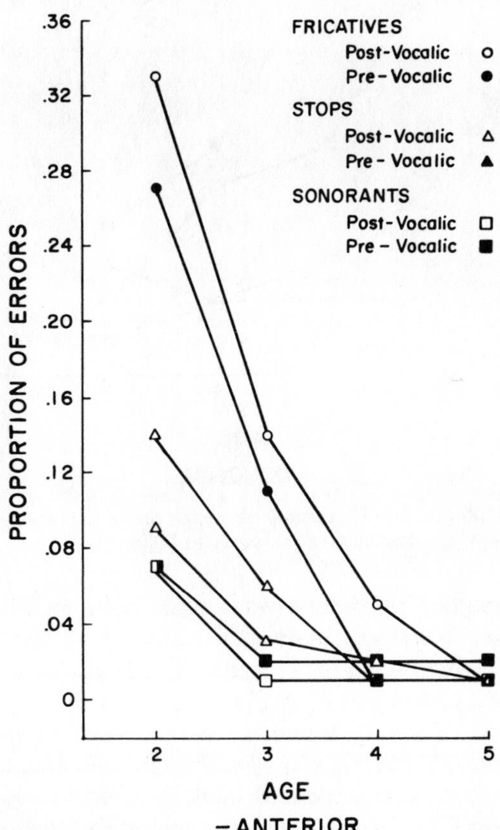

Figure 7-13. The proportion of −anterior errors for pre- and postvocalic fricatives, stops, and sonorants in children two to six years of age.

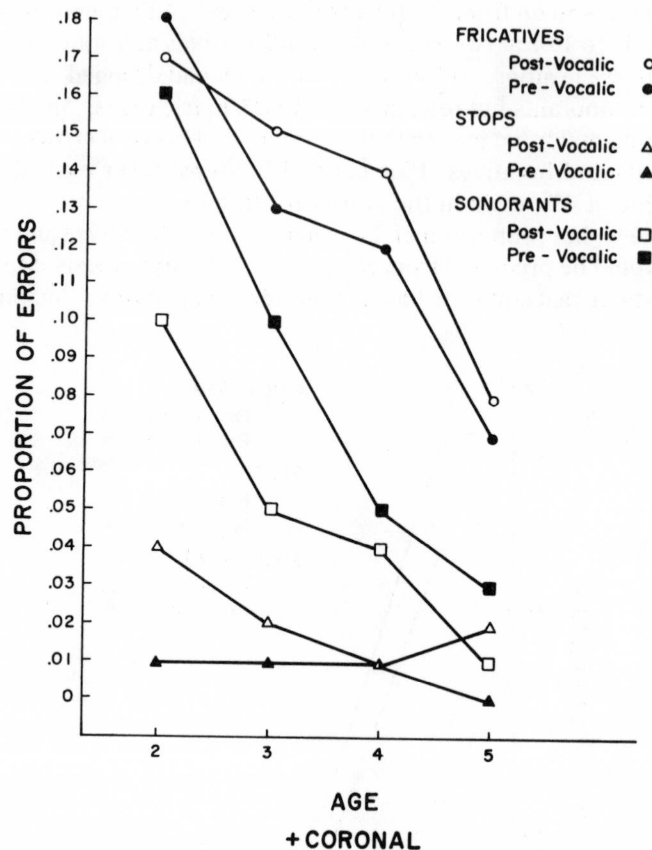

Figure 7-14. The proportion of +coronal errors for pre- and postvocalic fricatives, stops, and sonorants in children two to six years of age.

tions of the tongue'' other than what might be termed basic tongue positions. Plus coronal sonorants and fricatives include /r/, /s/, /z/, /ʃ/, /ʒ/, /θ/ and /ð/, which seem to involve tongue manipulations in which there are no anchor points for the tongue tip or blade.

Errors for −coronal during the production of pre- and postvocalic fricatives /f/ and /v/; stops /p/, /b/, /k/, and /g/; and sonorants /m/ and /ŋ/ (which only appeared in the postvocalic position) are shown in Figure 7-15. The only class of sounds that exceeded an error rate of 4% at any age tested was the postvocalic fricatives /f/ and /v/. This finding was expected, however, because the word-final position is generally acknowledged to be the most difficult context in which to produce an obstruent (Wise, 1958).

High The proportion of +high errors in stops /k/, /g/, /tʃ/, and /dʒ/; fricatives /ʃ/ and /ʒ/; and sonorants /w/, /j/, and /ŋ/ for each age level is represented in Figure 7-16. /ŋ/ was the only +high postvocalic sonorant and /w/ the only +high prevocalic sonorant. Errors on +high were instances where the tongue body failed to make palatal or velar contact when the idealized target sound called for such a contact. Errors on −high were instances where the tongue body made palatal or velar contact when the idealized target sound should have been

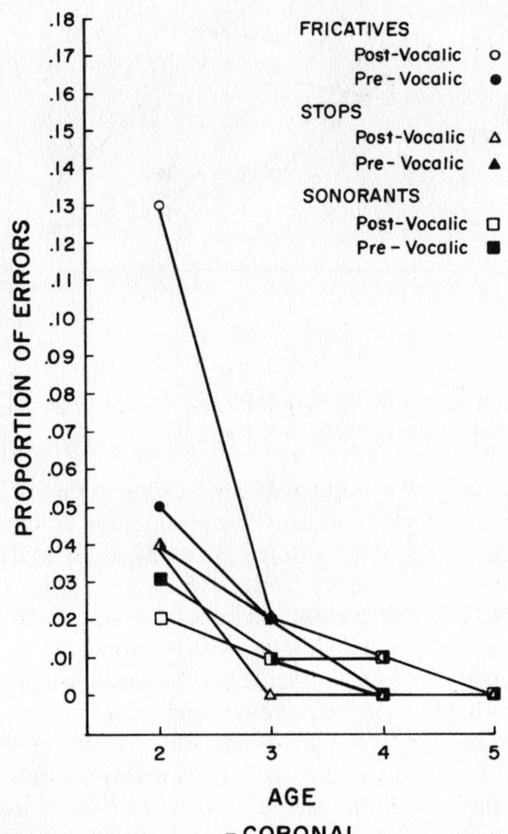

Figure 7-15. The proportion of −coronal errors for pre- and postvocalic fricatives, stops, and sonorants in children two to six years of age.

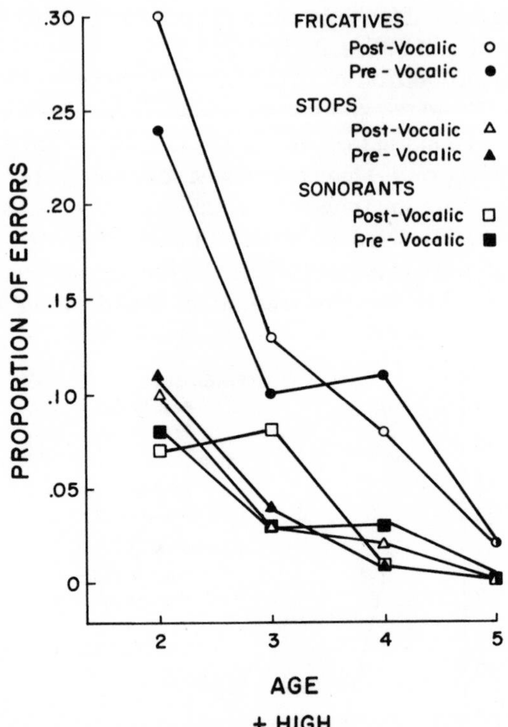

Figure 7-16. The proportion of +high errors for pre- and postvocalic fricatives, stops, and sonorants in children two to six years of age.

produced without such a contact. It can be seen in Figure 7-16 that at age two the +high feature during the production of sonorants and stops was in error 7 to 11% and fricatives 24 to 30%. By age four, +high was in error 3% or less except for fricatives, whose errors had declined to 8 to 12%. These results are also consistent with Menyuk's (1972) assertion that the last sounds to be mastered are those involving "tongue manipulations" other than the basic tongue positions. For example, +high in the fricatives /ʃ/ and /ʒ/ are produced without any anchor points while +high in /tʃ/ and /dʒ/ are produced with anchor points. Because the data points for fricatives represent only /ʃ/ and /ʒ/ (sounds without anchor points) in this figure, it is not surprising to see such a discrepancy between stops and fricatives.

The proportion of errors on −high in pre- and postvocalic stops /p/, /b/, /t/, and /d/; sonorants /r/, /l/, /m/, and /r/; and fricatives /f/, /v/,

/θ/, /ð/, /s/, and /z/ for each age level is presented in Figure 7-17. Sonorants (10% errors) were the only group of sounds with error rates that exceeded 4%. Close inspection of the data revealed that most errors in sonorants were attributable to a variant of /r/ that closely approximated /w/. The approximation of /w/ for /r/ is a common error in the prevocalic position but not in the postvocalic position (Van Riper and Irwin, 1958).

Back The proportion of +back errors in sonorants and stops for each age level studied is presented in Figure 7-18. /w/ was the only +back prevocalic sonorant and /ŋ/ was the only +back postvocalic sonorant. The +back stops /k/ and /g/ occurred in both pre- and postvocalic positions. Normally there are no +back fricatives in English.

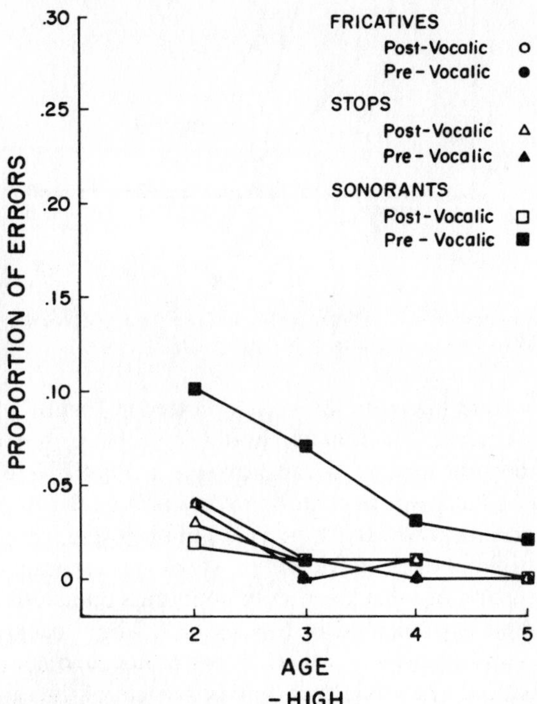

Figure 7-17. The proportion of −high errors for pre- and postvocalic fricatives, stops, and sonorants in children two to six years of age.

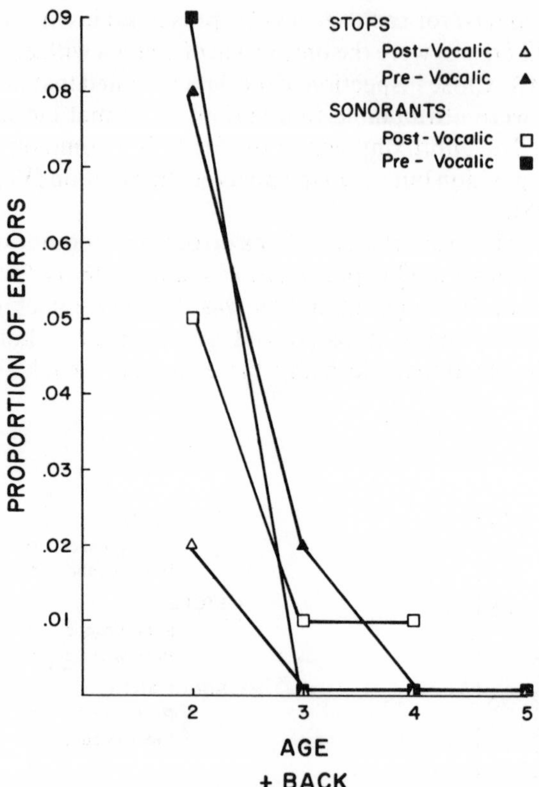

Figure 7-18. The proportion of +back errors for pre- and postvocalic stops and sonorants in children two to six years of age.

The proportion of errors for +back plotted in Figure 7-18 represents instances where the tongue should have been, but was not, retracted in the oral cavity. It can be seen in Figure 7-18 that for two-year-olds, +back was in error 8 to 9% in prevocalic stops /k/ and /g/ and 5% in sonorant /w/. By three years of age there were no more than 2% errors for +back in fricatives, stops, or sonorants.

The proportion of −back errors in sonorants and stops for each age level studied is presented in Figure 7-19. The −back pre- and postvocalic sonorants are /m/, /n/, /r/, /l/, with /j/ occurring only in the prevocalic position. The −back pre- and postvocalic stops are /p/, /b/, /t/, /d/, /tʃ/, and /dʒ/, and the −back pre- and postvocalic fricatives are /f/, /v/, /θ/, /ð/, /s/, /z/, /ʃ/, with /ʒ/ occurring only in the postvocalic position. Errors in Figure 7-19 represent instances where tongue retraction inappropriately occurred. The only error rate higher than 3% in −back occurred within prevocalic sonorants /l/, /r/, /n/, and /j/ for two-year-olds. In prevocalic sonorants −back was in error 7% of the time but was never in error at age five. Intuitively, the paucity of errors within −back was predictable because tongue retraction would demand more effort than tongue nonretraction. In other words, ease of production would predict that subjects would not use tongue retraction when this posture was not part of the target sound.

Distributed The proportion of +distributed errors in the pre- and postvocalic positions for each age level is presented in Figure 7-20. All sonorants and stops are +distributed. The +distributed fricatives include /s/, /z/, /ʃ/, and /ʒ/. Errors in Figure 7-20 represent

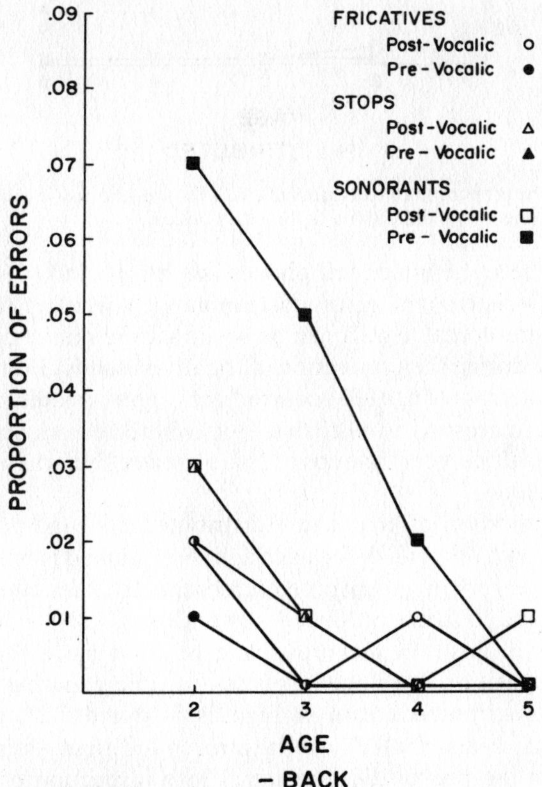

Figure 7-19. The proportion of −back errors for pre- and postvocalic fricatives, stops, and sonorants in children two to six years of age.

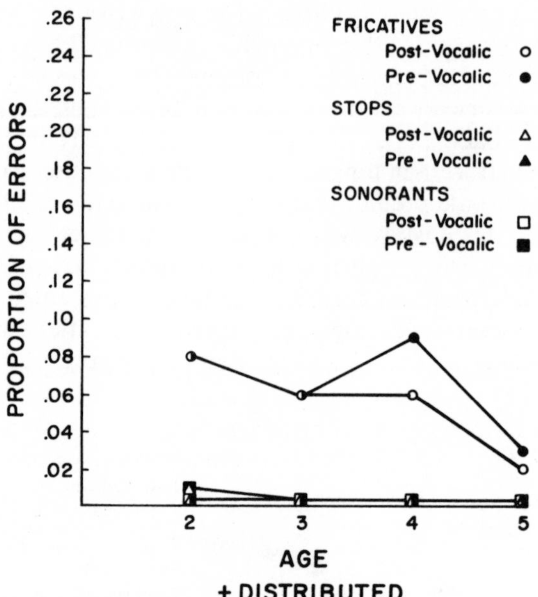

Figure 7-20. The proportion of +distributed errors for pre- and postvocalic fricatives, stops, and sonorants in children two to six years of age.

instances where the nondental phones /s/, /z/, /ʃ/, and /ʒ/ were dentalized. A +distributed error corresponds to what is frequently termed an interdental lisp. It can be seen that the only +distributed errors occur during the production of fricative sounds. Furthermore, +distributed errors of 6 to 8% occurred until approximately five years of age. It is interesting to note that +distributed errors plateau and persist over a three-year time span. This plateau effect was not seen in any other feature.

The proportion of errors in −distributed pre- and postvocalic fricatives /f/, /v/, /θ/, and /ð/ for each age level studied is presented in Figure 7-21. Errors in −distributed represent instances where dental /f/, /v/, /θ/, and /ð/ were produced as nondentals. The −distributed feature was in error in the prevocalic position more than in the postvocalic position at all age levels tested. In comparing +distributed and −distributed errors in Figures 7-20 and 7-21, it can be observed that −distributed was in error more than +distributed, especially in the prevocalic position. Close inspection of the data revealed that the majority of −distributed errors occurred in /θ/ and

/ð/. These sounds involve interdental articulations that are unique to relatively few languages. Because features that are universal are learned earliest (Jakobson, 1968), it is not unreasonable to expect a relatively unique articulation to result in a relatively high proportion of errors.

Nasal Figures 7-22 and 7-23 represent the proportion of +nasal and −nasal errors in sonorants, stops, and fricatives for each age level studied. The +nasal sounds are /m/, /n/, and /ŋ/ and all other sounds are −nasal. Errors on +nasal occurred when the velopharyngeal valve was closed during the production of /m/, /n/, or /ŋ/. Errors on −nasal occurred when the velopharyngeal valve opening was abnormally large. The sounds /m/ and /n/ occurred in the prevocalic position and /m/, /n/, and /ŋ/ occurred in the postvocalic position. As can be seen in Figures 7-22 and 7-23, there was less than 1% error on both +nasal and −nasal, even at two years of age. The proportion of errors on +nasal was the least for any of the features investigated with the exception of −lateral and −low. It can be inferred from these results

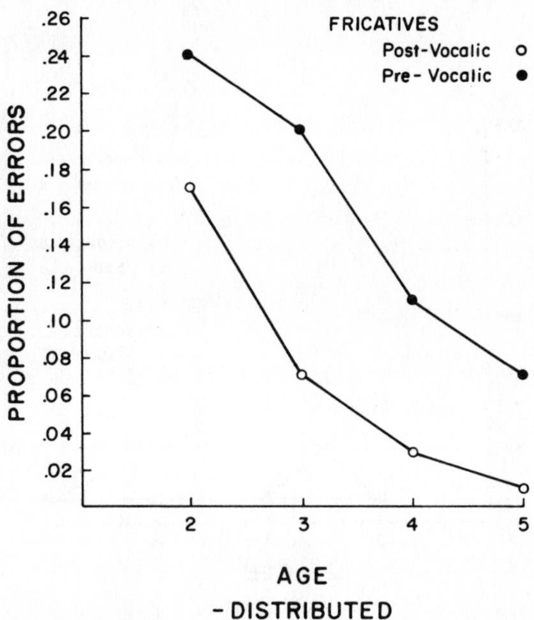

Figure 7-21. The proportion of −distributed errors for pre- and postvocalic fricatives in children two to six years of age.

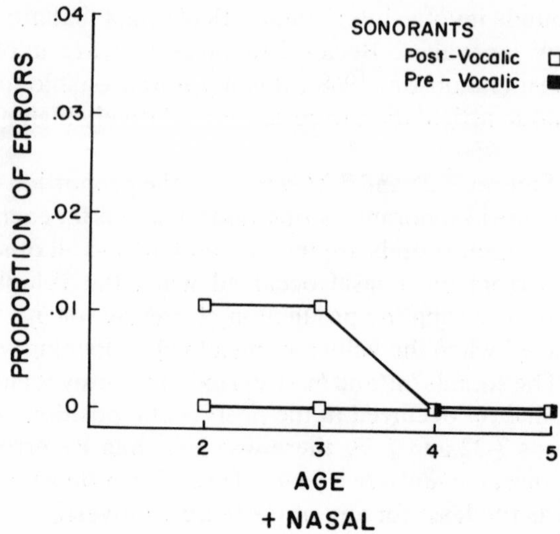

Figure 7-22. The proportion of +nasal errors for pre- and postvocalic sonorants in children two to six years of age.

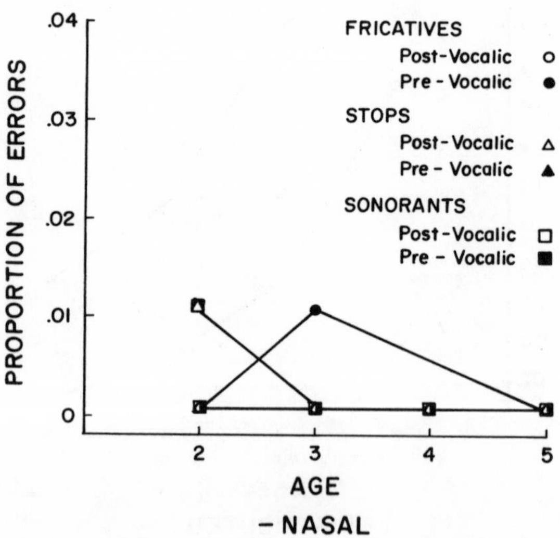

Figure 7-23. The proportion of −nasal errors for pre- and postvocalic fricatives, stops, and sonorants in children two to six years of age.

that the nasal distinction is acquired before two and a half years of age. Menyuk (1968) reported that +nasal was the first feature mastered of those she examined. She found 75% correct usage of +nasal for American children and about 95% correct usage of +nasal for Japanese children at two years, six months. The results of this present study support Menyuk's findings that +nasal is used correctly at two years, six months.

Lateral Figures 7-24 and 7-25 represent the proportion of +lateral and −lateral errors in the pre- and postvocalic positions for each age level studied. /l/ is the only phoneme in English that is +lateral. A +lateral sound is produced with the middle portion of the tongue lowered to allow a lateral escape of air; in nonlateral sounds (all other English phonemes except /l/), no such side passage is open for the air stream to flow out of the oral cavity. Figure 7-24 represents +lateral errors that occurred during /l/ productions. It can be seen that 7% or less +lateral errors occurred in the postvocalic position for all age

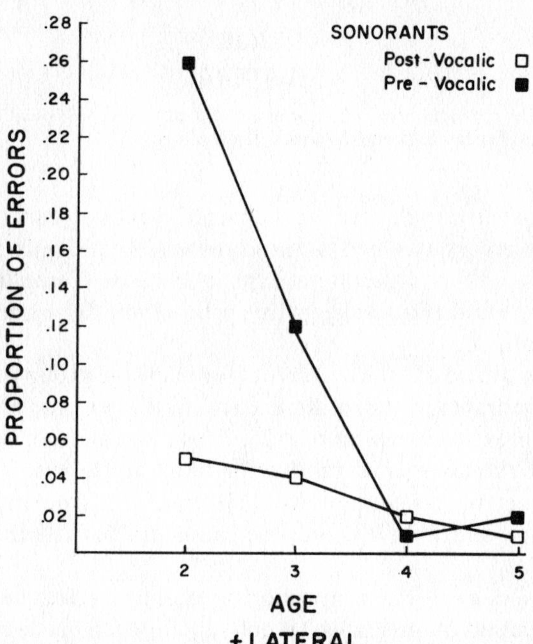

Figure 7-24. The proportion of +lateral errors for pre- and postvocalic sonorants in children two to six years of age.

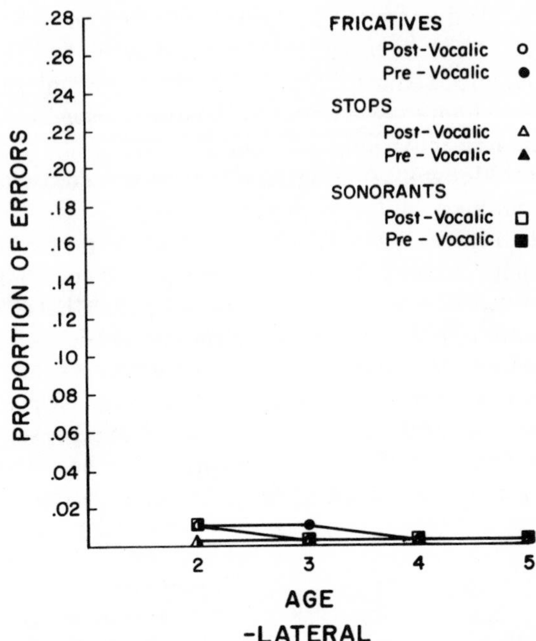

Figure 7-25. The proportion of −lateral errors for pre- and postvocalic fricatives, stops, and sonorants in children two to six years of age.

groups. In contrast, in the prevocalic position at two years of age, the proportion of errors was 26%, at three years 12%, and only 1% at four years. This result is difficult to explain because Templin's (1957) phoneme acquisition data suggest that postvocalic /l/ is acquired later than prevocalic /l/.

The proportion of −lateral errors for each age group during production of sonorants, stops, and fricatives in the pre- and postvocalic positions is presented in Figure 7-25. There were 2% or less errors regardless of the manner of production at all age levels. The higher proportion of errors on +lateral would be predicted from markedness theory because lateral in /l/ is marked and lateral for all other sounds is unmarked.

Delayed Release The proportion of +delayed release errors during the production of affricates /tʃ/ and /dʒ/ for each age level studied is presented in Figure 7-26. Affricates are the only phoneme class with +delayed release. Errors for +delayed release occurred when the articulators failed to produce a narrow passageway during the brief period immediately following release of the articulators.

In Figure 7-26 it can be seen that the proportion of +delayed release errors was 26 to 30% at two years of age, 8 to 11% at three years of age, and less than 5% at four years of age. Plus delayed release is sometimes considered a subfeature of −continuant because it occurs only in −continuant sounds. However, a comparison of the proportion of errors occurring on −continuant and +delayed release shows that the proportion of +delayed release errors was much greater than −continuant errors. Therefore, the majority of +delayed release errors had to occur while −continuant was maintained and must be considered independent of −continuant errors.

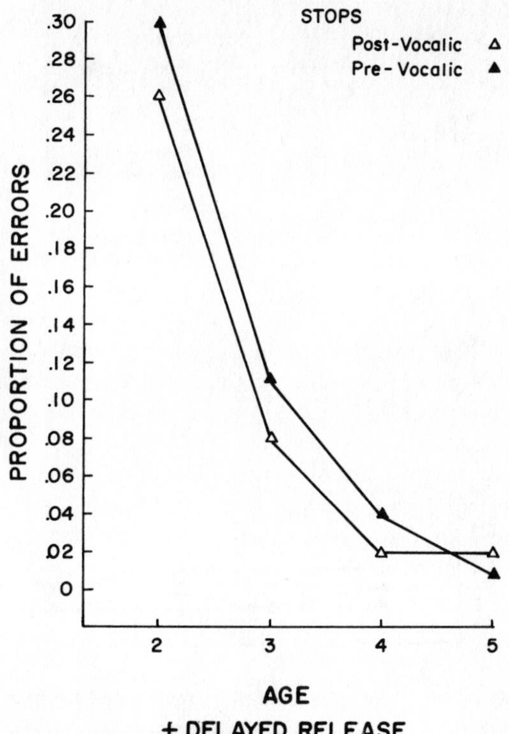

Figure 7-26. The proportion of +delayed release errors for pre- and postvocalic stops in children two to six years of age.

The proportion of −delayed release errors during fricatives, stops, and sonorants for each age level studied is presented in Figure 7-27. Errors for −delayed release occurred when fricatives, stops, or sonorants were affricated. As can be seen in Figure 7-27, less than 3% errors occurred for all ages studied.

Continuant The proportion of +continuant errors in the pre- and postvocalic positions for each age level studied is presented in Figure 7-28. The fricatives /f/, /v/, /θ/, /ð/, /s/, /z/, /ʃ/, and /ʒ/ and sonorants /m/, /n/, /ŋ/, /w/, /j/, /l/, and /r/ are +continuant. Plus continuant errors occurred when the breath stream was completely obstructed during the production of a +continuant. As can be seen in Figure 7-28, essentially no +continuant errors occurred within sonorants. At age two, an 8 to 16% error rate occurred for +continuant during the production of fricatives. By five years of age there were

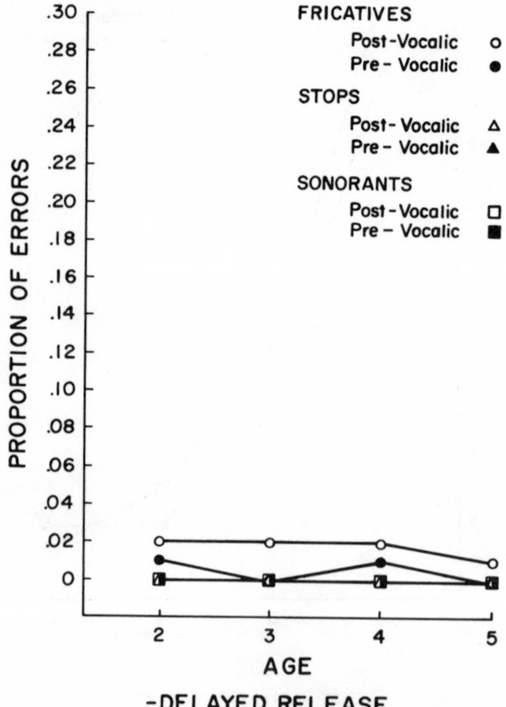

Figure 7-27. The proportion of −delayed release errors for pre- and postvocalic fricatives, stops, and sonorants in children two to six years of age.

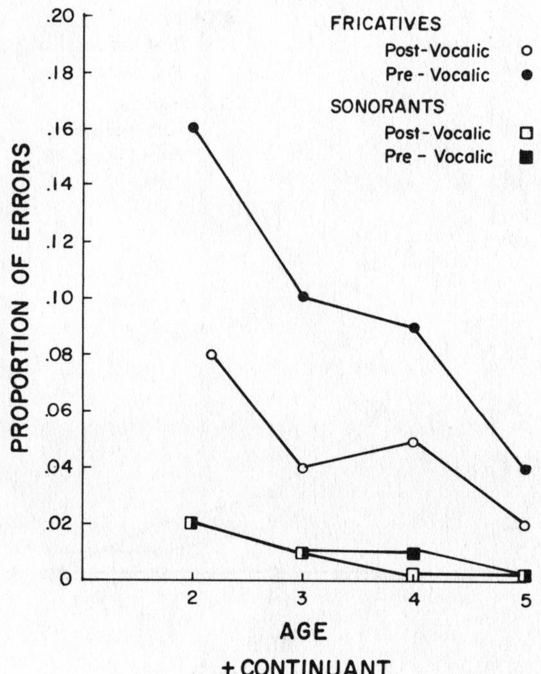

Figure 7-28. The proportion of +continuant errors for pre- and postvocalic fricatives and sonorants in children two to six years of age.

less than 5% +continuant errors in both pre- and postvocalic fricatives. Prevocalic fricatives resulted in more +continuant errors than did postvocalic fricatives.

Continuant is marked in fricatives and unmarked in stops and sonorants. Therefore, the higher proportion of +continuant errors in fricatives would be predicted from markedness theory. Substitution of stops for fricatives (unmarked for marked) is a common occurrence in children's speech (Van Riper and Irwin, 1958; Singh and Frank, 1972).

The proportion of −continuant errors within stops for each age level tested is presented in Figure 7-29. Stops and affricates /p/, /b/, /t/, /d/, /k/, /g/, /tʃ/, and /dʒ/ and sonorants /m/, /n/, and ŋ/ comprised the −continuant sounds. Minus continuant errors occurred when the breath stream was not completely impeded during a −continuant production. It can be seen in Figure 7-29 that −continuant in stops was in error 6% for two-year-olds and was less than 3% by three years

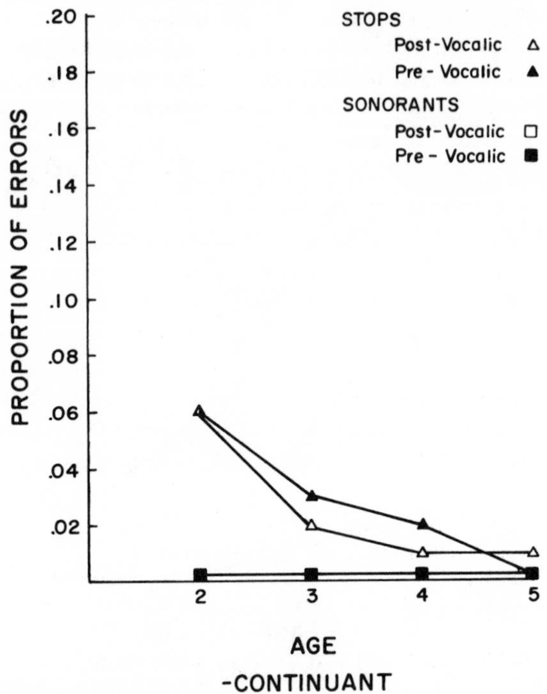

Figure 7-29. The proportion of −continuant errors for pre- and postvocalic stops and sonorants in children two to six years of age.

of age. Minus continuant in sonorants was always correct at every age level tested.

Voice The proportion of +voice errors that occurred during the production of pre- and postvocalic fricatives /v/, /ð/, /z/, and /ʒ/; stops /b/, /d/, and /g/; and sonorants /m/, /n/, /ŋ/, /r/, /j/, /l/, and /w/ for each age level studied is presented in Figure 7-30. Plus voice errors occurred when normally voiced sounds were produced in the absence of vocal fold vibration. Inspection of Figure 7-30 reveals that the majority of these +voice errors occurred during the production of fricatives /v/, /ð/, /z/, and /ʒ/ in the postvocalic position. At age two there were 17 to 27% +voice errors in fricatives and prevocalic stops. By age five, all +voice errors were 2% or below with the exception of postvocalic fricatives. Few +voice errors occurred during prevocalic stops or pre- and postvocalic sonorants.

Voiced obstruents form a natural class of voiced phonemes that behave differently from voiced sonorants. This distinction has been captured through the device of marking, wherein +voice in obstruents is marked and −voice in obstruents as well as +voice in sonorants is unmarked. Therefore, the greater magnitude of errors for +voice stops and fricatives supports the predictions of markedness theory.

The proportion of −voice errors that occurred during the fricatives /f/, /θ/, /s/, and /ʃ/ and the stops /p/, /t/, and /k/ for each age is presented in Figure 7-31. Minus voice errors occurred when sounds normally produced without vocal fold vibration were produced with vocal fold vibration. From Figure 7-31 it can be seen that relatively few −voice errors occurred within fricatives and stops, even at two years of age. These results would be expected because the replacement of voiced for voiceless would involve additional effort than normally would be demanded. In fact, analysis of children's errors rarely reveals substitutions of voiced for voiceless sounds.

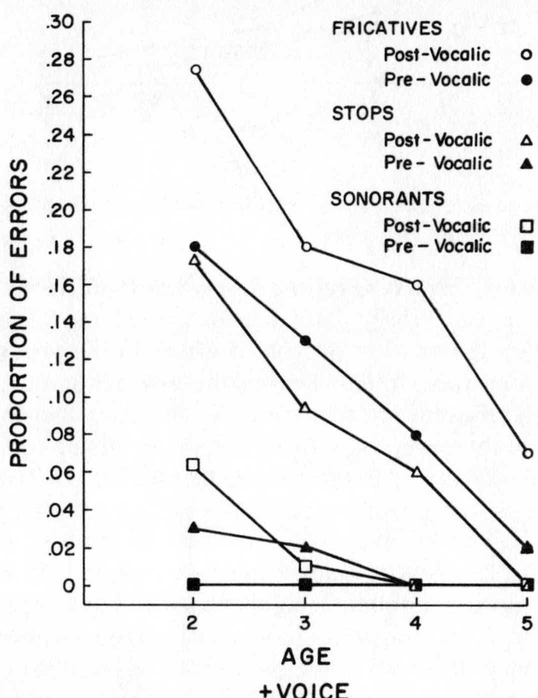

Figure 7-30. The proportion of +voice errors for pre- and postvocalic fricatives, stops, and sonorants in children two to six years of age.

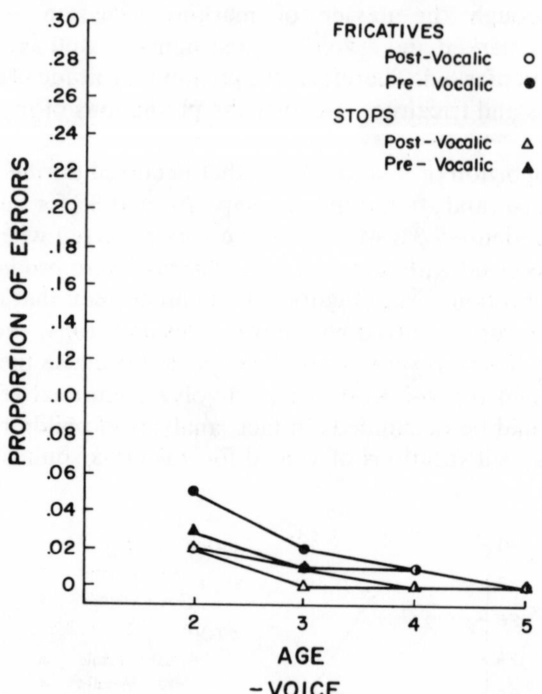

Figure 7-31. The proportion of −voice errors for pre- and postvocalic fricatives and stops in children two to six years of age.

Comparison of Errors in Pre- and Postvocalic Position Few significant differences (arbitrarily defined as differing by ≥ 5% at two age levels) between the number of feature errors in the pre- and postvocalic positions were found. During the production of fricatives, there were significantly more errors on +voice in the postvocalic positions while there were significantly more errors on −distributed and +continuant features in the prevocalic position. During the production of stops, there were significantly more +back errors in the prevocalic position while there were significantly more +voice errors in the postvocalic position. During sonorant production, there were significantly more +coronal, −high, +back, −back, and +lateral errors in the prevocalic position than in the postvocalic position. The higher frequency of errors in the prevocalic position for sonorants was unexpected because more misarticulations have been reported in the word-final position than in the word-initial position (Templin,

1957; Ervin-Tripp, 1966). However, Snow (1963) reported no differences between the number of misarticulations found in the word-initial and word-final positions. The equivocal results when comparing the number of feature errors between prevocalic and postvocalic positions would not support the notion that one can expect more sound errors in the postvocalic position.

Features with the Highest Proportion of Errors The identification of features that had the highest proportion of errors was determined by examination of the data collected from the two-year-old group. The reader should keep in mind that in this study the children labeled as the two-year-old group ranged in age from two years to two years, eleven months with a mean age of two years, seven months. Features were arbitrarily assigned a high difficulty rating when the feature was in error ≥ 10% in either the pre- or postvocalic position within a class of sounds, i.e., stops, sonorants, or fricatives. More features exceeded the criterion for a high difficulty rating during production of fricatives than during production of stops or sonorants. Features with a high difficulty rating during fricative productions were: −anterior, +coronal, −coronal, +high, −distributed, +continuant, and +voice. Features with a high difficulty rating for stops were: −anterior, +high, +voice, and +delayed release. Those with a high difficulty rating for sonorants were: +coronal, −high, and +lateral. The features of −anterior, +coronal, +high, and +voice received a high difficulty rating in at least two of the three sound classes examined in this study. It is interesting that three of these features, −anterior, +coronal, and +high, were place features.

Examination of the data from the oldest group studied (five-year-old group) revealed that only three features (+coronal, −distributed, and +voice) had an error rate that exceeded 5% in any sound class. The 5% error rate was exceeded only during the production of fricatives. It has been shown from sound acquisition data that, in general, correct production of fricatives is preceded by correct production of stops and most sonorants. These prior investigations obviously are in agreement with the present results, which showed that children between the ages of five and six years had more difficulty with the production of fricatives than with the production of stops or sonorants.

Markedness The results obtained from four of the eleven features investigated would have been predicted on the basis of markedness theory. The greatest number of anterior errors were on /ʃ/, /ʒ/,

/tʃ/, /dʒ/, /k/, and /g/ (−anterior fricatives and stops), which are marked for anterior. The phoneme /l/ is marked for the lateral feature, and so it was noted that the greatest number of errors occurred for /l/. Continuant is marked for fricatives, and the greatest number of continuant errors occurred within the fricative category. And finally, more errors were seen for +voice stops and fricatives, which are marked for voicing.

chapter 8
Distinctive Features in Articulation Deviation

CONTENTS

Haas (1963)
Elbert, Shelton, and Arndt (1967)
Crocker (1969)
Weber (1970)
Compton (1970)
McReynolds and Huston (1971)
Pollack and Rees (1972)
McReynolds and Bennett (1972)
Singh and Frank (1972)
Oller (1973)
Kamara, Kamara, and Singh (1974)
Kelly (1973) and Kelly and Singh (in preparation)
Compton (1975)
McReynolds, Kohn, and Williams (in press)
Costello (in press)

The basic elements of speech sound production are the distinctive features. Different systematic combinations of a relatively small number of distinctive features yield all the phonemes of a language. Distinctive features define phonemes and describe the interrelationships of different phonemes. On the one hand, they are the underlying bases of phoneme production, and on the other hand a measurable parameter of articulatory, acoustic, and psychological dimensions.

Articulation deviancy is mainly a disorder of distinctive feature misapplication in a particular phonetic environment. It is, therefore, only logical to describe phonemic deviancies in terms of distinctive features. In recent years, there have been a few experiments in which distinctive features have been the primary focus of interest in describing articulation problems, in planning articulation therapy, and in measuring the extent of progress made during the course of therapy.

HAAS (1963)

The articulation performance of a dyslexic 6.5-year-old male child was analyzed by Haas (1963). The consonant substitutions were analyzed by the articulatory features plosive, sibilant, nasal, liquid, and place of articulation. A comparison of the articulatory behavior of this child with standard English pronunciation revealed that distinctive features adequately accounted for the child's consonantal substitution errors. Haas concluded that the important element in teaching sounds of speech was the discrimination of those features that the child fails to produce: "In devising the most appropriate sequence of steps we shall take account of two things: (a) a gradation of English phonological distinctions according to their importance, and (b) another gradation according to difficulty the child may be expected to find in any of the distinctions it is to acquire" (p. 244).

ELBERT, SHELTON, AND ARNDT (1967)

Elbert, Shelton, and Arndt (1967) conducted an experiment to determine the transfer of training in seven subjects who had articulation problems. The consonants chosen for investigation in this experiment were /s, z, r/, which are some of the most commonly erred consonants in articulation disorder cases. The subjects were trained to produce correctly only the /s/ phoneme, with the hope that transfer would occur. Results for one of the seven subjects are plotted in Figure 8-1, which shows that the training on /s/ simultaneously improved the /s/ and /z/ phonemes but not the /r/ phoneme. The implication of these results is significant to both distinctive features and the morphophonemic aspects of English sounds. The fact that an exclusive training of /s/ simultaneously improves /z/ and not /r/ clearly demonstrates the acquisition of the distinctive features of /z/ via the distinctive features of /s/. These two phonemes share all features except voicing.

In addition, /s/ and /z/ are the most important entities for pluralizing English words. Thus, while learning the production of /s/, the subject perfects the pluralization rule. The pluralization rule may be learned as one entity; therefore, the Elbert, Shelton, and Arndt (1967) subjects improved significantly on both /s/ and /z/ items. The fact that /r/ did not show any improvements may result from the fact that, according to the distinctive feature count, the /s/ and /r/ phonemes are far apart. According to the distinctive feature system of Chomsky and

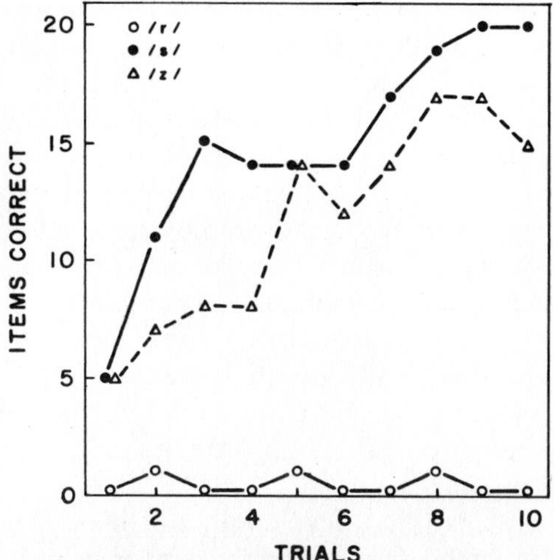

Figure 8-1. Scores for one subject's learning of phonemes /r/, /s/, and /z/ as a function of trials. Only the /s/ phoneme was worked with, with the hope that transfer of training would occur for the /z/ and /r/ phonemes. (From Elbert, Shelton, and Arndt, 1967; reprinted by permission.)

Halle (1968), the phonemes /s/ and /r/ differ by four features, and, according to the feature system proposed by Singh and Black (1966), these phonemes differ by five features. A large number of distinctive feature differences between the /s/ and /r/ phonemes intervened in the transfer of training between the two phonemes. To the contrary, the minimal distinction between the /s/ and /z/ phonemes was conducive to the transfer of training tasks.

CROCKER (1969)

Crocker (1969) has developed a model of children's consonantal phonological competence based on the distinctive feature models proposed by Chomsky and Halle and Jakobson, Fant, and Halle. He stressed the orderly and systematic nature of the child's competence throughout its emergence. He suggested that children do not learn individual phonemes or features per se but rather learn rules for combining features and classes of features to form new phonemes. "The [Crocker] model does not postulate that one sound is learned from another sound. It states, rather, that a feature is taken from an established feature set and combined with another feature to establish a new feature set or sound" (Crocker, 1969, pp. 206 and 208).

In outlining his model Crocker has divided Chomsky and Halle's distinctive features into three categories: primary, secondary, and cognate. The primary category is the most basic and includes the features vocalic, consonantal, nasal, and strident. The secondary category includes the features continuant, diffuse, voiced, and grave. The cognate category refers to the plus or minus specification of one feature; phonemes are called cognates if they are identical except for their values on the same feature (e.g., /p/ and /b/).

A "set" is defined as the combination of features that make up a phoneme. These sets may be similarly classified (again, from the most general to the more specific levels) into prime sets (the basic division of vocalic/consonant), base sets (from which further sets may develop), terminal sets (from which no further sets can develop), and derived sets (all others).

Crocker maintained that development of phonological competence may be adequately explained by these rules, which act upon the above feature sets. Like Jakobson, Crocker viewed development as proceeding from an undifferentiated general level to the specific level. Crocker's rules may be summarized by his statement: ". . . a child develops his phonological system by combining primary or secondary features with prime feature sets to form derived sets which may be base or terminal" (p. 206).

Both normal and deviant articulatory development may be explained by such a model. A sound may be misarticulated because of the complex combination of feature sets required for its mastery, because certain critical features were not mastered earlier in development, or because the sound was confused with one whose features appeared earlier in a different feature set. Errors of articulation, then, are not random but predictable from the feature sets and rules.

In conclusion, Crocker stressed that his model of systematic phonological development seemed to be substantiated by data from several well known studies.

WEBER (1970)

Weber (1970) studied the articulation and speech discrimination abilities of 18 children with articulation problems. Using the major features of place, manner, and voicing, Weber determined which features served a contrastive function (to yield phonemic classes) and which features served a noncontrastive function (to yield the allophonic variations). The analysis of errors of the major phonetic class features led Weber to conclude that several phonetic and phonemic errors are governed by patterns or rules involving distinctive features.

Having described the feature errors in the articulation and speech discrimination behaviors of his sample children, Weber established a therapeutic strategy aimed at features rather than consonants. The patterns or rules underlying the phonetic and phonemic errors ranged from one to six errors, with most children exhibiting two or three errors. The treatment was individualized depending on the pattern of error of each child. For example, one therapy was planned around the finding that a child's "manner feature contrasts were incomplete for stop/fricative, stop/semivowel, and stop/resonant. First the child was taught to discriminate auditorily between the manners in question, for example, between [t] and [s], [t] and [r], and [t] and [w]. Once he discriminated these contrasts auditorily, he was taught to produce them expressively" (p. 140). Weber's goal was to correct the deviant pattern and the features underlying the pattern rather than the individual phonemes. In his study, "the treatment was based on two main principles, which differed from the traditional approach to articulation therapy. (1) An entire pattern or category was taught at once rather than one sound at a time. (2) The child was taught to consciously contrast the incorrect feature with the correct feature throughout all stages of therapy" (p. 141).

COMPTON (1970)

Compton (1970) studied the articulatory substitutions of two children. He highlighted the role of distinctive features underlying the articulation problems. The focal points in his study were to emphasize some methodological advances made in the process of data reduction in the analysis of articulatory substitutions. In the Compton study, two major points of special interest to speech pathologists were that: 1) children's articulation errors are systematic, with the underlying elements in phonemic substitutions being the distinctive features, and 2) distinctive features are highly economical properties for the analysis of children's substitution patterns. For example, 12 phonological rules (Compton's Table 3) were necessary to describe one child's consonantal misarticulations in the initial word position. When distinctive feature analysis was introduced, the 12 rules were reduced to seven rules (Compton's Table 4). The use of distinctive feature principles in describing misarticulations not only economizes the process of description but also provides a more exact account of the phonological principles underlying the substitutions.

Upon completion of the distinctive feature analysis of two patterns of children's misarticulation, Compton concluded that: "The defective sounds of speech characterizing an articulatory disorder are part of a coherent and productive system organized by means of phonological principles" (p. 339). What appears, on the surface level of speech production, to be an extensive problem of articulation in fact may be only a misapplication of a small number of underlying rules. Once the underlying distinctive feature rule is clarified, all surface level misarticulations would be corrected to the desired model. Jim, one of the two children in the Compton study, exhibited two problems with his nasal consonants: unusual lengthening of the final nasals /m, n, ŋ/ and the accompanying release into the oral stops. Therapy was concentrated exclusively on the /m/ phoneme, with the assumption that, if the misarticulations of the final nasals were three different surface representations (/m, n, ŋ/) of one underlying distinctive feature, nasality, then a change in the total performance of all nasal consonants could be effected by working with the one feature, nasality.

The result was consistent with the hypothesis that the lengthening of nasal consonants stemmed from one feature error. Compton wrote that: "of the total 17 final-nasal consonant items included in the test (five for /m/, six for /n/, and six for /ŋ/, with at least two repetitions of each), there was not a single occurrence of the earlier misarticulations of any of the nasal consonants, even though therapy had been limited only to /m/" (p. 337). Thus, it was the use of the feature that was erred and the use of the feature that needed to be corrected. The distinctive features, on the one hand, revealed the exact nature of the underlying problems with each of the phonemic misarticulations and, on the other hand, served as a clear basis for therapy. Although distinctive features, as an underlying system in phoneme productions, are abstract entities, their psychological, articulatory, and acoustic realities have been verified. Thus, distinctive features serve as an important tool to relate the phonological and phonetic domains.

McREYNOLDS AND HUSTON (1971)

McReynolds and Huston (1971) investigated the problem formulated by Compton (1970) that a few underlying distinctive feature problems may account for a much greater number of misarticulated consonants. They investigated whether a feature misarticulated in one phoneme was also misarticulated in other phonemes containing the feature. They also examined the hypothesis that a feature absent in the phoneme where it belongs may appear in the phoneme where it does not belong.

The results of their experiment are best illustrated in their two figures that show the plottings of the phonemic misarticulations and the distinctive feature errors of the same child. Figures 8-2 and 8-3 are taken from McReynolds and Huston to show the magnitude of phonemic misarticulations and the magnitude of the distinctive feature errors. Figure 8-2 is the plotting of consonant and vowel misarticulations of one subject. It shows that 15 of the 28 speech sounds were misarticulated over 50% of the time. A subsequent inspection, shown in Figure 8-3, found that none of the distinctive features was erred over 50% of the time and that only the plus specifications of the features continuancy, voicing, stridency, high and back were erred over 20% of the time. The plotting of feature errors shows that the distinctive features responsible for most of the consonant misarticulations were continuancy, voicing, and back. In addition, only the plus specifications of these features contributed to most of the consonant misarticulations.

A close examination of Figure 8-3 also reveals that the plus specification of the features vocalic, consonantal, nasality, continuancy, voicing, stridency, coronal, high, and back, and the minus

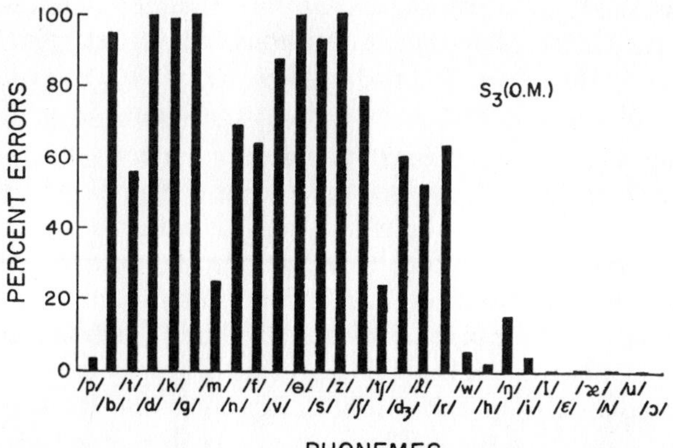

Figure 8-2. Percentage of errors made by one subject (subject 3, O.M.) for individual phonemes. (From McReynolds and Huston, 1971; reprinted by permission.)

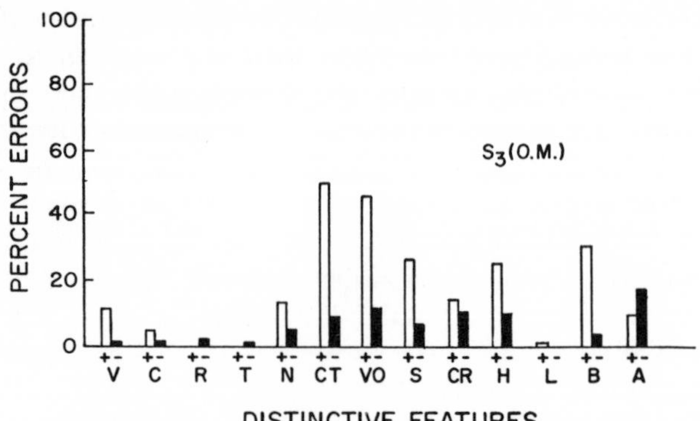

Figure 8-3. Percentage of errors made by one subject (subject 3, O.M.) on plus and minus specifications of 13 Chomsky and Halle features. V, vocalic; C, consonantal; R, round; T, tense; N, nasal; CT, continuant; VO, voicing; S, stridency; CR, coronal; H, high; L, low; B, back; and A, anterior. (From McReynolds and Huston, 1971; reprinted by permission.)

specification of the feature anterior, contributed to most of the misarticulations in the subject's production of the test material. According to markedness theory, the plus specifications of those features that contributed to the greatest number of errors are marked (M) whereas the minus specifications are unmarked (U). For example, +continuancy, +voicing, +stridency, +high, and +back are marked feature specifications. For the feature anterior, however, it is the minus specification that is considered marked. Consistent with the notion of markedness, −anterior accounted for more errors than +anterior. It may be recalled that a marked feature specification implies greater articulatory complexity than its unmarked counterpart. It is hypothesized, therefore, that markedness of features is a valid measure for predicting distinctive feature errors of consonants.

Ten children tested by McReynolds and Huston (1971) with the McDonald Deep Test had a wide range of phonemic misarticulations. On the average, over 80% of the time the 10 children mispronounced 10 of the 28 phonemes tested. However, on the average they only made errors on 1.3 features of the 13 features employed. Figure 8-4 is a plotting of percentage of features used by the 10 children against the features present in the McDonald Deep Test. These percentages have been extrapolated from Table 2 in McReynolds and Huston (1971). This figure shows that the 11 Chomsky and Halle features applicable to the consonants were rank ordered. The features used the greatest number of times were coronal, low, and consonantal, and the features used the fewest number of times were stridency, voicing, and continuancy. For most of the features, the poorest subject was subject 1 and the best subject was subject 10. The remaining subjects fell between these two. Figure 8-4 also shows that all features were not misarticulated equally, and that some features were misarticulated the least by all 10 subjects. For example, the features coronal, low, consonantal, back, high, and anterior showed better performances than the features vocalic, nasality, stridency, voicing, and continuancy.

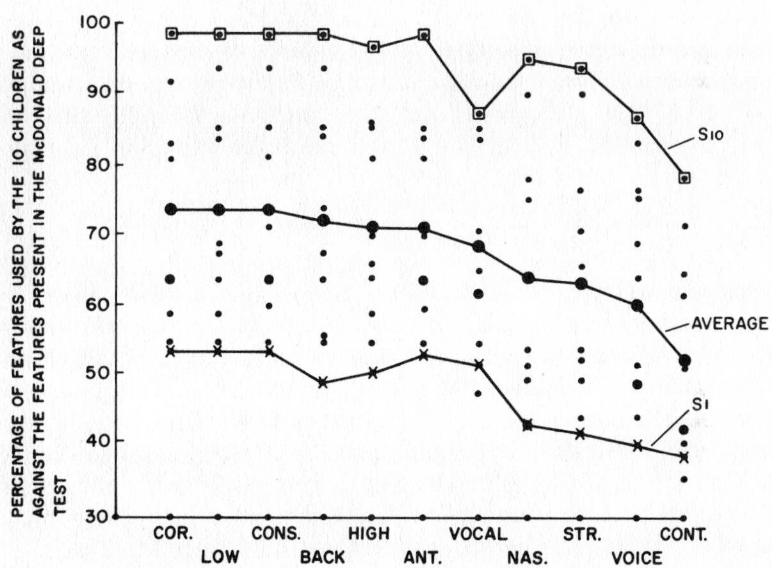

Figure 8-4. Percentage of features used by the 10 children against the features present in the McDonald Deep Test. The points for the best, the worst, and the average subjects have been connected. (Reanalysis by Singh of McReynolds and Huston, 1971.)

POLLACK AND REES (1972)

Distinctive feature analysis of the articulation disorder of a male child was performed when the child was five years, two months; five years, eight months; and six years, three months. During this one-year period the child was in therapy. Adult norms were used as reference points for the child's speech. Any deviancy in articulation from the adult norm was considered a misarticulation. The substitution inventory of phonemes was examined by two transcribers and subjected to a distinctive feature analysis involving the features voicing, nasality, continuancy, stridency, grave, diffuse, vocalic, and consonantal (Halle, 1964).

At age five years, two months, child B.N. made two feature substitutions (gravity and diffuseness) resulting in six phonemic substitutions. Twelve consonants were omitted, indicating the absence of both the plus and minus specifications of continuancy, voicing, nasality, gravity, and diffuseness. At the final stage of therapy (age six years, two months), however, most substitutions were incorporated into the adult phonemic system. The essence of the feature training and feature analysis was summarized by Pollack and Rees: "A comparison of B.N.'s responses over three times of testing show how his system changed, maintaining an internal orderliness, but gradually approximating that of the adult model" (p. 456).

McREYNOLDS AND BENNETT (1972)

McReynolds and Bennett (1972) tested the feature generality hypothesis discussed earlier in Compton (1970). The generalization of three features across phonemes was tested in three children. First, the Chomsky and Halle (1968) feature system was used to analyze the consonant misarticulations of a group of children. These children and their error patterns have been described in McReynolds and Huston (1971). Three of the 10 children described earlier were chosen for distinctive feature training. A feature was used in training in the context of nonsense words. The features were taught first with the consonant at the initial position and then at the final position of a word.

The programmed steps in this study were as follows: The child learned to produce the plus or minus specification of a feature, whichever was absent in his repertoire, via a given phoneme. The child would learn to contrast the plus and minus specifications of a feature in a discrimination task. The contrast of the criterion phoneme was presented in the context of several vowels. The procedure was repeated for both initial and the final consonants of a syllable. A step of training was considered complete only if a child accomplished 90% correct accuracy. The training was concentrated on those features whose phonemic correlates were erred in the child's production. For example, if stridency was the misarticulated feature, the children were trained with one or two strident consonants, and after the criterion score was achieved they were probed for their learning of the remaining strident consonants /f, v, s, z, ʃ, ʒ/.

One of the three children whose performance was poor on the stridency feature was trained with /f/. Another child was trained for +voicing in the context of /b/. A third child was trained for +continuancy with the phoneme /ʃ/. The result of this three-feature training with the help of the token phonemes was very encouraging. The before training errors for the five strident consonants tested were 100%. The after training errors for that feature involving the same consonants were reduced to 20%. In order to determine whether the improvement was limited only to the +stridency feature, a control consonant, /θ/, was tested before and after the stridency training. The error was 100% at the base line and 100% after the final probe. The +voicing error before the voicing training with phoneme /b/ was 98% and after the training was reduced to 14%. Again, the control phoneme /θ/ showed 100% misarticulation both before and after training. Finally, the training with the phoneme /ʃ/ for the +continuancy feature resulted in a reduction of misarticulations from 100% to 31%.

In conclusion, it was proved decisively in this experiment that feature generalizations are a valid means for improving phonemic misarticulations. The method is highly economical and elegant because the emphasis is to rectify the *system* rather than the individual sounds. Because one feature is a component of several sounds, if that feature is established in the context of one sound, all other sounds bearing that feature are automatically corrected.

SINGH AND FRANK (1972)

Singh and Frank (1972) analyzed consonant articulation problems in 90 children whose mean age was 72.4 months and who exhibited normal hearing and neurological development. The substitutions for the "true" English consonants in these data were evaluated in light of a distinctive feature model. The matrix in Table 8-1 shows the features of consonants included for analysis in this study. The substitutions were counted for all children in the initial, medial, and final word positions. The results indicated that no phoneme is immune to substitution, yet not all phonemes are used as substitutes.

Table 8-1. The "true" consonant phonemes of English

	Labial	Interdental	Alveolar	Back
Nasal	m		n	ŋ
Stop	p, b		t, d	k, g
Fricative	f,v	θ, ð	s, z	ʃ, ʒ

Manner Substitutions

Within the manner of articulation category, the feature stop replaced the features nasal and fricative, but the feature fricative replaced neither nasal nor stop. Of the 311 manner substitutions, 299 were substituted by stops and the remaining 12 by nasals. An examination of the discrete articulatory events involved in producing the nasal consonants clearly shows why stop/nasal and stop/fricative substitutions are made, and why nasal/fricative substitutions are not made. Stop/nasal substitutions are made because they share oral occlusion, and stop/fricative substitutions are made because they share a lowered velum; nasal/fricative substitutions are not made because neither feature is shared:

	Nasal	*Stop*	*Fricative*
Velum lowered	+	−	−
Oral occlusion	+	+	−

Place Substitutions

The results pertaining to the place of articulation substitutions show that the place feature is substituted by the closest, more fronted place in the same manner series: in the stop and nasal series, alveolar for back and labial for alveolar, and, in the fricative series, alveolar for back, interdental for alveolar, and labial for interdental. The feature labial is not replaced because there is no place more fronted than labial. Thus, labial fricatives and labial nasals cannot change the place of articulation and can only change manner. Labial stops cannot change according to the rules for either the place or the manner substitutions.

Place and Manner Substitutions

If the closest fronted feature of place that normally would be used as a substitute is not yet available in the child's repertoire, there is a change in manner of articulation.

Principles Governing the Substitutions

The principle underlying the above substitution rules is a combination of phonemic "stability" and interphonemic "similarity." A feature is considered stable if it is substituted relatively infrequently. The earlier a feature is acquired, the more stable it is and the more likely that it will replace less stable features. However, stability alone does not explain the entire substitution pattern. Distinctive feature similarity between the substitute and the substituted phoneme plays an important role. An erred phoneme is usually replaced by the phoneme it is most similar to in terms of distinctive features.

Conclusions

On the basis of the distinctive feature analysis of 90 children with articulation problems, Singh and Frank (1972) drew the following conclusions:

1. The most recently acquired phonemes are replaced most often.
2. Phonemes used as substitutes are most often the ones learned earliest.
3. The stop feature is the most frequent replacement for other manner features:
    a. Fricatives and nasals are replaced by stops.
    b. Stops are not replaced.
    c. Nasals and fricatives do not substitute for each other.
4. A place feature is substituted by the closest more frontal place in the same manner of articulation:
    a. Alveolar replaces back.
    b. Interdental replaces alveolar.
    c. Labial replaces alveolar.
5. If the closest, more frontal feature has not yet emerged in the same manner series, then there is a change in both the place and the manner series. For example, according to rule 4a, /ʃ/ is replaced by /s/. However, if /s/ has not appeared in the child's repertoire, /ʃ/ is replaced by /t/.

6. Voiceless more frequently substitutes the voiced feature than vice versa.
7. Substitutions are influenced by stability and similarity of phonemes.

OLLER (1973)

Oller (1973) investigated the application of generative phonology to the speech sound substitutions of five abnormally speaking children. On the basis of positing both the phonemic level and the distinctive feature level rules, Oller demonstrated the economy and the succinctness of the distinctive feature rules over the phonemic rules. A total of 223 phonemic rules were considered essential to describe individually the misarticulations of the five children. In comparison, a total of 76 distinctive feature rules were required to account for the misarticulations of the same five children. The ratio of phonemic to distinctive feature rule was approximately 3:1.

In addition to the obvious economy, a number of generalizations regarding the articulatory system of the abnormal child were made in this study that would not be possible in the framework of phonemic analysis. A much greater regularity was found when an articulation disorder was examined by a distinctive feature system (Chomsky and Halle, 1968) than when it was examined by the phoneme as an ultimate analytic unit. These regularities suggest that children with articulation problems possess considerable competency in formulating phonological rules. An articulation therapist who gains insight into these rules can successfully transfer them to fit the appropriate norm.

KAMARA, KAMARA, AND SINGH (1974)

Kamara, Kamara, and Singh (1974) reported results from 77 children who represented a broad variety of populations referred to a southeastern Ohio speech and hearing clinic. These children's consonant substitution errors were obtained with the Kamara-Kamara-Singh Articulation Test of Distinctive Feature Competence (Kamara, Kamara, and Singh, 1974). Twenty-five consonant phonemes were tested in the three word positions. The substitutions, distortions, and omissions were analyzed utilizing a distinctive feature system described in Singh and Polen (1972) and Singh and Singh (1972b).

The notion of applying distinctive features to describe both articulation and speech discrimination errors was proposed by Singh

(1973). The repeated emergence of distinctive features in both speech perception and speech production research was the main reason for devising a reliable distinctive feature system for use in diagnosis. The data reported in Chapters 5, 6, and 7 of this book support the notion that distinctive features are utilized for both articulatory and discriminatory commands and, therefore, can describe both articulation and speech discrimination problems

A "feature-gram" is the plotting of a subject's speech discrimination and/or articulation scores in terms of distinctive features. In a typical feature-gram, the distinctive features are presented in a fixed order on the abscissa and the percentage of correct articulation and/or speech discrimination scores is presented on the ordinate. A subject's unique feature-gram profile proves to be extremely useful for evaluation and therapy. Although a number of distinctive feature systems can be used with reasonable predictive accuracy (Wang and Bilger, 1973), the feature system used by Kamara, Kamara, and Singh (1974) included a binary set of seven distinctive features: front/back place, labial place, sonorancy, nasality, continuancy, sibilancy, and voicing.

After the feature-grams for each of the 77 subjects were plotted, a statistical technique was employed for grouping these subjects according to the profiles of their feature-grams. A stepwise discriminant analysis was used to group the subjects into their diagnostic categories. The 77 subjects fell into five groups: 1) pathology, lesion, organic group, 2) retarded group, 3) cleft palate group, 4) functional group, and 5) specific learning disability group. The discriminant analysis showed that this grouping was statistically significant.

Five feature-gram profiles were then plotted based on only those subjects' scores which were grouped by the discriminant analysis. Thus, the feature-gram for the pathology group was based on an *n* of five, the feature-gram for the mental retardation group was based on an *n* of four, the feature-gram for the cleft palate group was based on an *n* of three, the feature-gram for the functional articulation disorders group was based on an *n* of 30, and the feature-gram for the specific learning disability group was based on an *n* of six.

Figures 8-5 to 8-9 are the feature-gram profiles of pathology, retardation, cleft palate, functional disorders, and specific learning disabilities groups, respectively. The difference in the profiles of the articulation problems of these five groups of subjects is evident. In the first group, the profile shows a steady loss at all seven features. None of the feature scores exceed 50% correct level. The second group

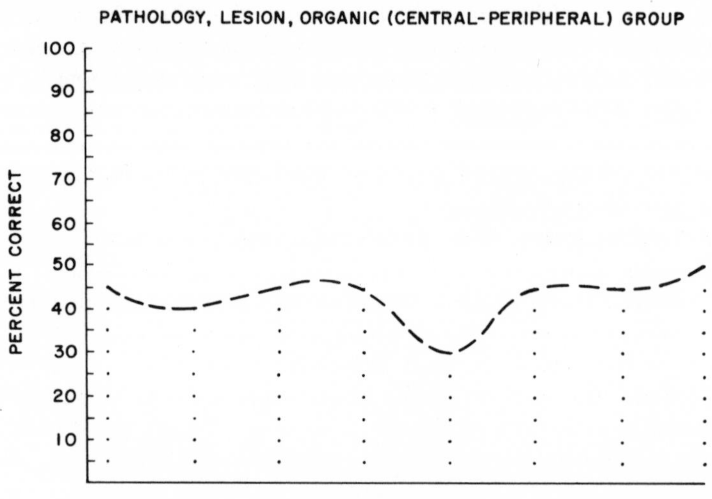

Figure 8-5. Production of percentage of correct feature for the pathology, lesion, organic group. (After Kamara, Kamara, and Singh, 1974.)

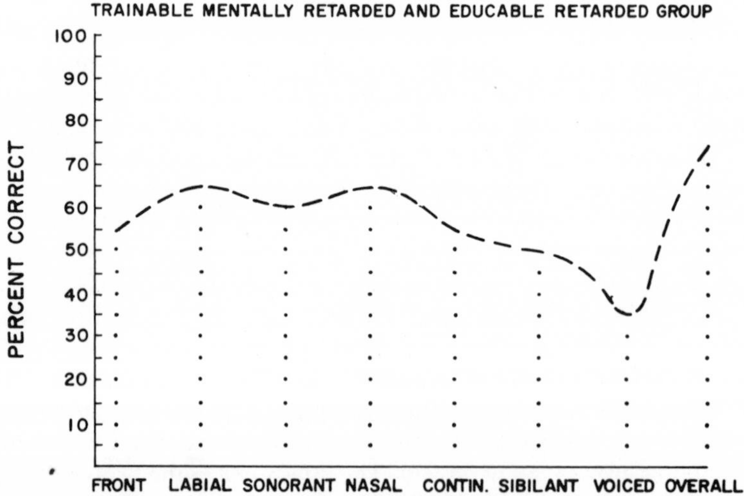

Figure 8-6. Production of percentage of correct feature for the trainable and educable mentally retarded group. (After Kamara, Kamara, and Singh, 1974.)

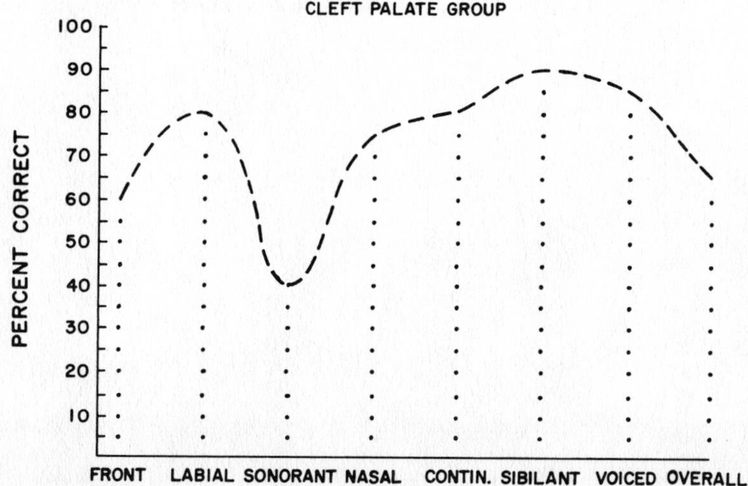

Figure 8-7. Production of percentage of correct feature for the cleft palate group. (After Kamara, Kamara, and Singh, 1974.)

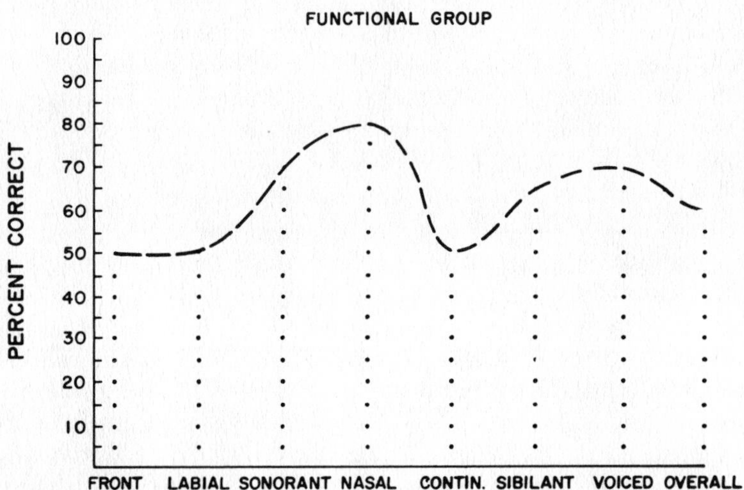

Figure 8-8. Production of percentage of correct feature for the functional disorders group. (After Kamara, Kamara, and Singh, 1974.)

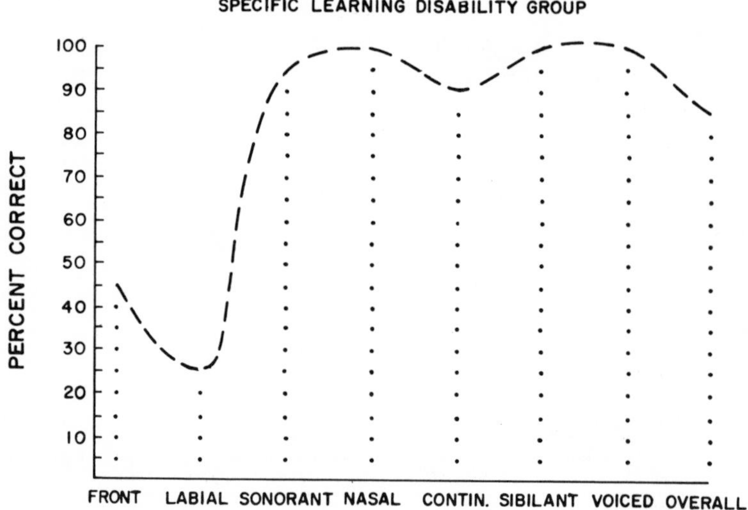

Figure 8-9. Production of percentage of correct feature for the specific learning disability group. (After Kamara, Kamara, and Singh, 1974.)

(mental retardation) shows a considerable dip at the voicing feature. The third group (cleft palate) shows greater than 70% scores for all features except front/back place and sonorancy; the maximal dip is on the sonorancy feature. The fourth group (functional disorders) shows poor scores for the place of articulation (front/back and labiality) and continuancy features, and better scores for the features nasality and sonorancy. Finally, the fifth group (specific learning disabilities) shows a significant dip at the features front/back place and labiality with practically no loss at any other features.

In summary, the pathology, lesion, organic group shows a low profile across all features; the retardation group shows low profile on the feature voicing; the cleft palate group shows a low profile on sonorancy; the functional group shows a low profile on place and continuancy; and the specific learning disabilities group shows a low profile on the place of articulation feature. Each of the five groups has a significantly different profile. This information is extremely useful for the diagnosis and therapy of the various articulation problems. Once the patient is appropriately classified into a diagnostic category, the clinician has an adequately established base line for planning clinical work.

KELLY (1973) AND KELLY AND SINGH (IN PREPARATION)

Kelly (1973) and Kelly and Singh (in preparation) studied the articulation problems of 60 children who ranged in age from eight to ten years. Thirty of these 60 children were normal and 30 had articulation problems. The Templin-Darley Diagnostic Test of Articulation (Templin and Darley, 1969) was used to select 60 subjects to constitute two groups. A score of 127 on the 141-item Templin-Darley Diagnostic Test of Articulation was used as the cutoff score for dividing these children into normal and defective articulation groups. A score of 127 was one standard deviation below the mean for eight-year-old boys and girls (Templin and Darley, 1969).

The phonetic substitutions of the 30 subjects who exhibited articulation problems were subjected to distinctive feature analysis using the system described in Singh and Polen (1972) and Singh and Singh (1972b). Although these children were all tested on the 141-item Templin-Darley test, the distinctive feature analysis was performed only on those 22 English consonants which appeared at the initial, medial, and final positions of a word. The question asked in this experiment was: What relationship exists between the Templin-Darley phonemic test scores, based on 141 items, and the distinctive feature scores (front/back place, labiality, sonorancy, nasality, continuancy, sibilancy, and voicing), based only on the substitution scores of 22 consonant items of the Templin-Darley test?

Results were analyzed by multiple regression. The Templin-Darley test scores on each of the 30 children with defective articulations were predicted by the 14 plus and minus specifications of each of the seven distinctive features noted above. The principal objective of applying stepwise multiple regression analysis was to determine the relative degrees of predictive power of each of the 14 specifications of the distinctive features. Because there were no errors made in the feature category +nasal, this category failed to yield any correlations. The outcome of the regression of the remaining 13 feature specifications on the Templin-Darley Test scores is shown in Table 8-2. This table shows that the order in which the variances were accounted for by these feature specifications was: back, nonlabial, voiced, sonorant, sibilant, continuant, nonsibilant, and front. The F ratios associated with the multiple R values and the t ratios associated with the contribution of each of these features individually were significant at the 0.01 level. Although the F ratios pertaining to the remaining feature variables—stop, labial, voiceless, non-nasal, and nonson-

Table 8-2. Multiple correlation coefficients, *F* ratios, and *t* values between Templin-Darley test scores and distinctive features for subjects with defective articulation

df	*R*	*F* ratio	*t* test
1,28	0.738	33.47[a] (back)	16.42[a]
2,27	0.801	24.17[a] (nonlabial)	7.29[a]
3,26	0.843	21.30[a] (voiced)	6.43[a]
4,25	0.881	21.63[a] (sonorant)	6.58[a]
5,24	0.889	18.07[a] (sibilant)	3.11[a]
6,23	0.900	16.36[a] (continuant)	3.73[a]
7,22	0.913	15.64[a] (nonsibilant)	4.04[a]
8,21	0.922	14.87[a] (front)	3.59[a]
9,20	0.925	13.24[a] (stop)	2.17
10,19	0.929	11.93[a] (labial)	2.16
11,18	0.929	10.35[a] (voiceless)	0.77
12,17	0.929	8.97[a] (non-nasal)	0.36
13,16	0.930	7.85[a] (nonsonorant)	0.74

[a]Significant at the 0.01 level.

orant—were significant, the individual t test was not significant. Thus, these feature specifications did not contribute significantly to the variance in the data.

The results of the multiple correlation and stepwise regression analyses between the seven distinctive features and the Templin-Darley test scores indicate that distinctive features can be used to predict performance on the Templin-Darley test with a high degree of reliability. Table 8-2 shows that the best predictor of the Templin-Darley test scores was the feature back. The correlation coefficient was 0.738 with a significant F value of 33.47 and a significant t value of 16.42. Table 8-2 also shows that the features back, nonlabial, voiced, sonorant, sibilant, continuant, nonsibilant, and front place jointly yield a correlation coefficient value of 0.992. Because each of these features has a significant F value and a significant t value, it may be concluded that they jointly and independently made significant contributions toward explaining almost all the variance in the data.

Because either none or insignificant errors were made in the feature categories of stop, labiality, voiceless, non-nasal, and non-sonorant, these features did not account for any significant amount of variance in the data. These features are very stable and rarely are the basis for articulation errors.

Figure 8-10 shows the plotting of three of the 30 subjects of the Kelly (1973) experiment. One subject had high Templin-Darley scores (123 of 141 possible), another subject had a below average score (111 of 141 possible), and the third subject had the lowest score (66 of 141 possible). The purpose of these plottings is to show some discrepancies between the Templin-Darley measure, which is based mainly on phonemic performance, and the distinctive feature measure, which reflects the underlying system. Except for +labiality, the subject performing below average on the Templin-Darley test scored 100% for all features. The subject with the high Templin-Darley score, however, exhibited less than perfect feature scores for −front, −labial, +labial, +continuant, −sibilant, and −voice. The subject with the poorest Templin-Darley test score showed serious problems only on −front, −continuant, and +sibilant features. All other feature scores of this subject were in the vicinity of 80% correct or higher. It may be noted that the feature scores were derived from the subset of the Templin-Darley test involving the use of consonants at the initial and final places. In conclusion, while the Templin-Darley score is a unitary measure of the patient's articulation performance, the distinc-

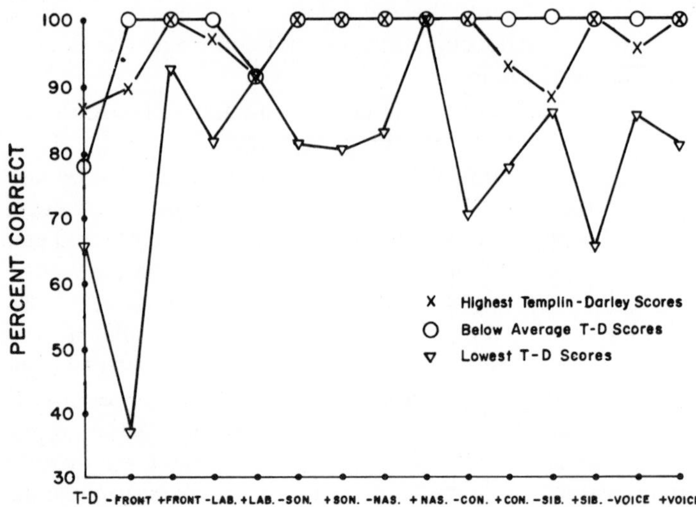

Figure 8-10. Plotting of percentage of correct feature scores for three subjects: one with a high Templin-Darley score, one with a below average Templin-Darley score, and the one with the lowest Templin-Darley score.

tive feature score is a measure of differential skill on a number of parameters reflecting the patient's underlying competence.

COMPTON (1975)

Compton (1975), in another study, applied distinctive feature principles to phonological rules to: 1) describe children's misarticulations, 2) make clinical applications of the distinctive feature principles, 3) propose normal developmental strategies, 4) show the relationship between normal and deviant phonological development, and 5) propose a theory of the acquisition of phonological disorders.

Use of Distinctive Features in Children's Misarticulations

Although the English language has about 45 phonemes, the parameters to describe them are less than one-fourth that number. Compton has proposed a distinctive feature system that includes six binary features and one feature, the place of articulation, with six values. He has applied this feature system to the interpretation of children's deviant articulation patterns.

Features are more economical to use in therapy because they reveal the multiple relationships between phonemes of a language.

Working with a single feature, a therapist might be simultaneously working with several speech sounds. Thus, for example, the feature voicing can be corrected by working only on one pair of consonants with the voicing contrast alone. The feature voicing would be correctly generated for seven other pairs of voiced/voiceless pairs of consonants.

The feature system proposed by Compton was selected arbitrarily. However, his reason for departing from his earlier reliance on the Chomsky and Halle (1968) feature system was that: "the feature system presented here is motivated mainly by very practical considerations concerned with explicitly describing normal and abnormal speech of children in the most simple and straightforward way possible" (p. 66).

Compton presented a phonological analysis of a five-year-old child named Frank to demonstrate the important procedural framework of an intensive distinctive feature analysis. Frank's speech was 80% unintelligible. He had an above average IQ with no physical or auditory problems. On an articulation test devised by Compton, Frank made extensive errors of the initial and final consonants and initial consonant blends of English. A tabulation of Frank's substitution errors showed that he made a much greater number and variety of errors at the final position than at the initial position of a word. For example, all stops, nasals, and sonorants were fairly well established at the initial position of the words. However, at the final position, there was a large number of substitutions. Frank's production of double and triple initial consonant clusters showed the tendency of reducing them to a single phoneme.

An inventory of the total misarticulations of Frank's consonants and consonant clusters showed that he made a total of 59 different substitutions of the underlying consonants, most of which were recurring. Eleven different substitutions were made at the initial consonant position and 24 different substitutions at the initial consonant cluster position. Twenty-four different substitutions were made at the final consonant position. Compton wrote 12 distinctive feature rules to account for the 35 initial position errors and seven distinctive feature rules to account for the 24 final position errors. Distinctive features are the inherent elements supporting the formulations of these phonological rules. For example, rule 1 is written as:

$$\begin{bmatrix} \text{stop} & + \\ \text{place} & 4 \\ \text{voice} & \pm \end{bmatrix} \rightarrow \begin{bmatrix} \text{stop} & + \\ \text{place} & 6 \\ \text{voice} & \alpha \end{bmatrix}$$

which indicates that /t/ → /k/ and /d/ → /g/. This rule is very efficient because it specifies every distinctive feature whether or not it is misarticulated. The only error in this particular example is a place of articulation error, which is specified as alveolar becoming velar. Thus, this rule does not only state the fact that /t/ → /k/ and /d/ → /g/ but also that /p/, /b/, /k/, and /g/ are correctly produced stops. Of course, there are other rules that implicate the problems of these phonemes as well as some other problems with the /t, d/ phonemes in Frank's misarticulations.

Clinical Applications of the Distinctive Feature Principles

Having derived the underlying principles of the variety of recurring misarticulations, a clinician can work with the various features in error. Once these features are established, they can be applied to all consonants and consonant clusters contrasted by that particular feature. Thus, in order to change the status of 59 different misarticulations in Frank's speech, a clinician may have to work maximally with 19 distinctive feature rules.

There were six reevaluation periods in the Compton study: *session 1* after 20 therapy sessions, *session 2* after 16 therapy sessions, *session 3* after 19 therapy sessions, *session 4* after 25 therapy sessions, *session 5* after 16 therapy sessions, and *session 6* after 24 therapy sessions. These therapy sessions were all designed to concentrate on the distinctive feature principle. Before each evaluation period, certain rules were chosen to be worked with and the clinician worked at those and only those rules.

Figure 8-11 shows the amount of success in correcting error rules (ordinate) preceding each of the reevaluation periods (abscissa). At the first reevaluation (after 20 therapy sessions), Frank had two of the 19 rules corrected. There were other rules that had changed but not totally normalized. At the second reevaluation period (after another 16 therapy sessions), seven rules had been totally corrected. Again, there were some other rules that had changed. At the third reevaluation period, nine of the 19 error rules had been perfected. At the fourth, fifth, and sixth reevaluation periods 12, 13, and 17 error rules, respectively, had been corrected. Thus, at the sixth reevaluation period only two rules, both optional and partially corrected, remained to be corrected. It must be emphasized at this point that the correction of error rules at each reevaluation period related very closely to the criterion rules chosen for work at the preceding therapeutic session. According to Compton: "The case study of Frank illustrates the

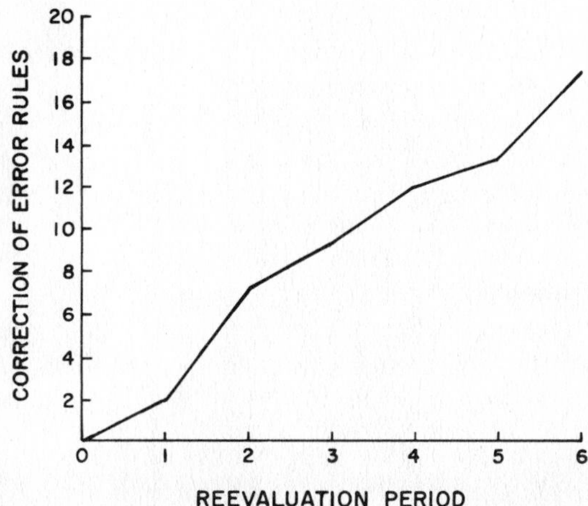

Figure 8-11. Correction of error rules as a function of reevaluation periods.

general strategy for translating a phonological analysis into a motivated plan for therapy. . . . the analysis itself is not a recipe for therapy. Rather, it is more like a map to aid us in choosing the best route to reach a destination'' (p. 87).

Normal Developing Phonological System

Having reported the success in converting Frank's 19 error rules to almost normal phonological behavior for a five- to six-year-old child, Compton provided some highlights of his hypothesis regarding normal phonological development. His conclusions were based on longitudinal study ''of the normal acquisition of speech, beginning with the first meaningful utterances at about 1 year and extending through the 3rd year, the age at which most children have fairly well mastered the sound system of their language'' (p. 87). His conclusion is consistent with distinctive feature theory: Children do not acquire phonemes one by one; rather, they acquire a feature that provides them with a basis for manifesting a number of phonemes distinctively in speech production and discrimination tasks.

Relationship Between Normal and Deviant Phonological Development

On the basis of the longitudinal study of phonological development of one- to three-year-old children, on the one hand, and the deviant phonological patterns of Frank and two other children described earlier (Compton, 1970), on the other, Compton showed a significant parallel between the normal and deviant articulation acquisition patterns. He listed eight general developmental trends that apply to both populations; e.g., the first syllable uttered is a consonant-vowel syllable, the first consonants are voiceless stops, the first fricative consonants are voiceless fricatives, greater substitutions occur across the category of place of articulation than across the category of manner of articulation, and so on.

A Phonological Theory

Compton (1975) proposed a number of postulates which he called "a theory of the acquisition of phonological disorders." His postulates can be summarized as follows:

1. Phonological disorders of an older child, e.g., five to six years of age, parallel the phonological indices of a younger normal child, e.g., a two-year-old.
2. The reason for the first postulate is that: "A child acquiring speech normally goes through various stages of omission and sound substitution patterns that are subsequently dropped or replaced by others as he moves from one phase of development to the next. The child with defective speech, however, seems to be operating according to some sort of rigidity principle by which he hangs on to and thus accumulates these patterns of omissions and substitutions which otherwise would be discarded in moving from one stage to another" (pp. 89–90).
3. The phonological principles underlying the disordered speech are not "primitive" or simplified but well developed and innovative.

McREYNOLDS, KOHN, AND WILLIAMS (IN PRESS)

McReynolds, Kohn, and Williams (in press) investigated the speech discrimination and production performances of seven children who made articulation errors of six or more phonemes. Seven normal children were also included in this study to compare the discrimination performance. The focal point of the study was to test whether or not children who misarticulate speech sounds also have a problem in discriminating them. The criteria for testing these children were six of the 13 Chomsky and Halle (1968) features. The features included for testing were: continuancy, nasality, voicing, stridency, anterior, and coronal. The articulation errors were determined by McDonald Deep Test items, and the discrimination scores were obtained by contrasting 80 minimally distinct pairs of consonants. These 80 pairs were generated by the six distinctive features. Subjects in the discrimination task were asked to press one of two buttons to signify same or different pairs of consonants.

The normal and the misarticulation groups performed at the same level in the discrimination task. There was a considerable difference, however, between the articulation and the speech discrimination scores of the misarticulation group. It may be concluded, therefore, that the only difference between the seven normally speaking children and the seven children who misarticulated was in their production of distinctive features and not in their discrimination abilities.

The results of this experiment may be interpreted in two ways: 1) that discrimination precedes production (Singh and Frank, 1972), and 2) that feature discrimination in a same/different task paradigm may not be investigating these children's decoding ability. An identification task, for example, may show that children with poor articulation performance also may exhibit poor identification performance.

COSTELLO (IN PRESS)

Costello (in press) has presented a procedure for applying distinctive features (Singh and Polen, 1972) in measuring articulation problems and in planning treatment. The utilization of distinctive feature principles in the description of articulation problems proved economical and effective. A comparison of the misarticulated consonant with the target phoneme revealed that 13 different phonemic substitutions could be accounted for by three distinctive features: 1) continuancy, 2) sibilancy, and 3) front/back place. Thus, in order to effectively treat the 13 incidences of phonemic substitutions, a speech pathologist need work with three features only. Costello concluded that such treatment procedures are not only effective, but are more efficient in terms of the number of phonemes modified in a given amount of instruction time.

The primary goal of reviewing the literature in this chapter is to demonstrate the efficiency of distinctive feature theory in the diagnosis and treatment of articulation problems. Although there has been a limited number of studies that directly test the relevance of distinctive feature theory in the treatment of articulation disorders, the available data heavily support the efficiency of this system on both diagnosis and treatment procedures.

chapter 9
Distinctive Features in Auditory Discrimination

CONTENTS

Singh (1968): prediction of multiple choice intelligibility tests by a distinctive feature system
Tannahill and McReynolds (1972): same/different discrimination task
Singh and Blackmon (1974): Modified Rhyme Test
Singh, Lawson, and Singh (1974): Modified Rhyme Test
Danhauer and Singh (1975c): feature-gram study
Some other experiments: casting doubt on distinctive feature theory

The role that distinctive features play in the perception of consonants and vowels has been well established and amply described in Chapters 5 and 6 of this text. We have evidence that it is the knowledge of distinctive features that a listener invokes in perceiving consonants and vowels. Although there has been a considerable number of experiments conducted in the area of speech perception to substantiate the above statement, very little effort has been made to apply distinctive features in the prediction of speech discrimination tests. Because distinctive feature research dealing with phoneme perception shows that it is the distinctive feature of a phoneme that listeners utilize in perception, the speech discrimination tests, mostly designed to assess the hearing-impaired individual's speech perception, need to be interpreted by distinctive features.

SINGH (1968): PREDICTION OF MULTIPLE CHOICE INTELLIGIBILITY TESTS BY A DISTINCTIVE FEATURE SYSTEM

The listeners' errors on a multiple choice intelligibility test (Black, 1957) were predicted by a distinctive feature system (Singh and

Black, 1966). This test requires a listener to identify on a printed answer sheet a word from a group of four similar sounding words. The group of four words comprised a stimulus word and three decoy words. The disparity between the correct response, i.e., the stimulus word, and the actual response, i.e., the response selected from one of the three decoy words, was measured in terms of the number of distinctive feature differences.

The distinctive feature analysis of the error responses of the multiple choice intelligibility tests shows a linear relationship, with almost a direct correlation between the number of errors among words and their distinctive feature differences. This finding is extremely encouraging for those who need to apply distinctive features in diagnosing the auditory processing of speech stimuli. The feature system applied here was arbitrarily selected, yet the correlation was very high. Similarly, the Modified Rhyme, Consonant-Nucleus-Consonant, and Connected Speech Tests (Singh, Faircloth, and Faircloth, in press) also show high correlations in a variety of speaking and listening conditions.

TANNAHILL AND McREYNOLDS (1972): SAME/DIFFERENT DISCRIMINATION TASK

Tannahill and McReynolds (1972) determined the role of distinctive features in the auditory differentiation of consonants. Forty-five pairs of consonants were presented to listeners with the opposition of consonants in a given pair controlled by the Miller and Nicely (1955) feature system. The subjects were to indicate whether or not the consonants in a given pair were the same or different. The discrimination task was made more difficult by passing the stimuli via a lowpass filter. The analysis of the results revealed that greater confusions occurred when the consonants of a pair were contrasted at zero- and one-feature difference levels than when contrasted at two-, three-, and four-feature difference levels. Figure 9-1 shows the plotting of the mean percentage of errors associated with the different levels of distinctive feature difference. Except for levels 2 and 3, all other levels yielded significantly different consonant confusion scores. The final conclusion obtained in this experiment was: "that discrimination of consonant pairs was differentially affected by the number of opposing features contained in each pair. Further, as the numbers of opposing features increased from 0 to 4, percentage of errors decreased significantly" (p. 108).

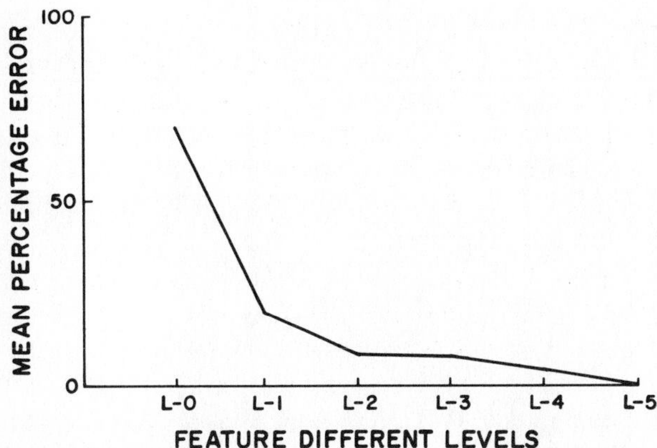

Figure 9-1. Mean percentage of errors as a function of different levels of distinctive feature differences of consonants.

SINGH AND BLACKMON (1974): MODIFIED RHYME TEST

The purpose of the Singh and Blackmon (1974) study was to make a distinctive feature prediction of the errors that listeners made on the Modified Rhyme Test (House et al., 1965). The listeners were 25 college students with normal speech and hearing performances. Three speaker lists of Modified Rhyme Test stimuli were presented under signal-to-noise conditions that yielded 83% discrimination (high) and 75% discrimination (low) scores.

A distinctive feature analysis of the Modified Rhyme Test was performed before the experiment. A multiple comparison for each of the 50 Modified Rhyme Test items was based on distinctive feature differences among the six words in each item. There were 15 different distinctive feature relationships within each item ($6 \times 5 \div 2 = 15$), or 750 for the entire Modified Rhyme Test ($50 \times 15 = 750$). The results of this analysis appear in Table 9-1. Column 1 in this table shows the distinctive feature differences ranging from zero to seven feature differences. Column 2 shows the number of comparisons in the Modified Rhyme Test associated with each of these differences. For example, in the Modified Rhyme Test there are 138 pairs of words differing by one feature, 178 pairs of words differing by two features, and so on. Figure 9-2 is the plotting of distribution of the 750 word pairs in the Modified Rhyme Test. This figure is based on the values presented in Table 9-1. It shows that most word pairs in the Modified

Table 9-1. Distinctive feature analysis of the Modified Rhyme Test

Feature differences	Number of word pairs in Modified Rhyme Test associated with feature differences
1	138
2	178
3	182
4	174
5	65
6	11
7	2
Total	750

Rhyme Test are different from each other by two, three, and four features. Figure 9-3, taken from Singh (1970b), plots English consonants as they relate to each other according to the distinctive features. Comparison of these two figures suggests that the Modified Rhyme Test and English in general share a similar distribution of distinctive feature differences. Thus, the Modified Rhyme Test seems a valid instrument for investigating speech discrimination ability.

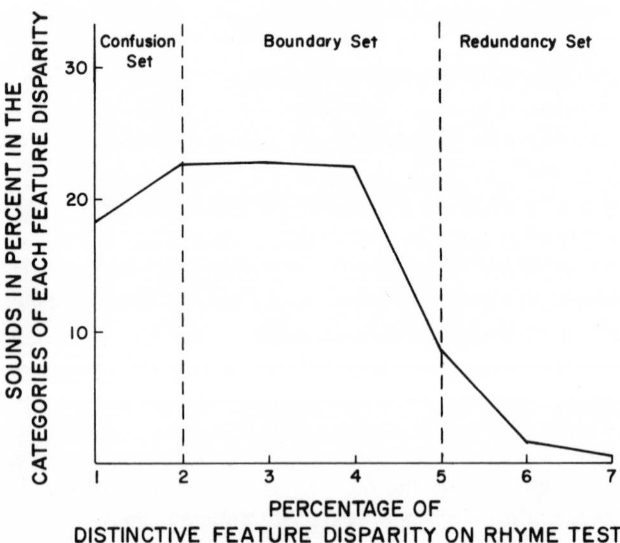

Figure 9-2. Number of consonants in one to seven feature categories. The sample was limited to Modified Rhyme Test stimuli.

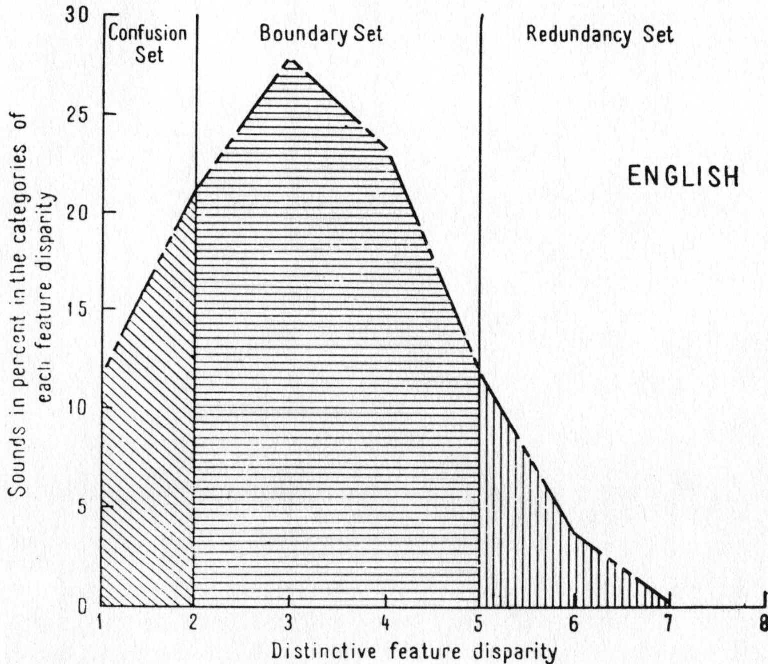

Figure 9-3. Number of consonants in one to seven feature categories for the phonemic system of the English language. (From Singh, 1970a.)

The final goal of this study was to predict the Modified Rhyme Test error scores by the 25 listeners using a distinctive feature system (Singh, Woods, and Becker, 1972). It was hypothesized that the greater the feature difference between the stimulus and response words of the Modified Rhyme Test, the fewer the number of errors. Figure 9-4 is the plotting of the weighted distribution of errors made by subjects for all speaker (three) and performance (two) conditions. The abscissa in this figure shows the distinctive feature difference, and the ordinate shows the error scores weighted by the frequency of occurrences within each feature category. A nearly perfect correlation was obtained between the number of errors between the stimulus word and the response word, and the distinctive feature difference between them.

SINGH, LAWSON, AND SINGH (1974): MODIFIED RHYME TEST

The study by Singh, Lawson, and Singh (1974) is an extension of the earlier experiment by Singh and Blackmon (1974). Modified Rhyme

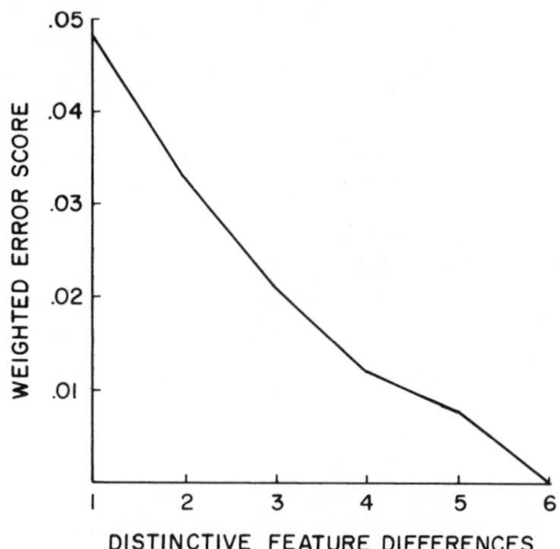

Figure 9-4. Weighted distribution of errors made by all subjects for all speaker conditions of the Modified Rhyme Test.

Test scores of 30 subjects who were referred to hearing and speech clinics for hearing evaluations were predicted by the distinctive features of the consonant phonemes. These subjects were given pure tone threshold tests, speech reception threshold tests, and Modified Rhyme Tests 1 and 2. The total number of right ears tested was 25 for lists 1 and 2, and the total number of left ears tested was 24 for lists 1 and 2. Thus, there was a total of 98 confusion matrices resulting from the 49 ears and two list conditions. The confusion matrices were the results of the subjects' listening errors on the Modified Rhyme Test stimuli.

The main goal of this experiment was to group the 98 confusion matrices according to their diagnostic categories. The experimenters had three sets of scores on each subject and each ear: 1) pure tone test results, 2) speech discrimination test results, and 3) the results from the distinctive feature analysis of the phonemic discrimination errors.

A stepwise discriminant analysis technique described earlier in Chapter 8 (Kamara, Kamara, and Singh, 1974) was employed to determine the diagnostic groupings inherent in the 98 confusion matrices. First, the pure tone audiogram results were correlated with the distinctive feature profiles. The results showed that only 30 of the 98 cases grouped according to pure tone losses were confirmed by the distinctive feature profiles. However, the stepwise entry of the seven distinctive features to predict the pure tone audiogram scores showed no significant *F* ratio. Next, speech discrimination results were correlated with the distinctive feature profiles. Of the total 98 possibilities, the grouping of 66 subjects was predicted by the distinctive feature profiles. The stepwise entry of the distinctive features revealed significant *F* ratios for the features voicing, sibilancy, and sonorancy. Although this result was more encouraging than the one dealing with the prediction of pure tone audiogram scores, 32 of the 98 confusion matrices remained unpredicted.

In the third stage of the analysis, therefore, the 98 confusion matrices were grouped by one of the seven distinctive feature scores and predicted by the total distinctive feature profiles. The result of one such analysis is presented here.

The feature labiality was chosen to group the 98 confusion matrices into five groups. The groups were formed by the percentage of correct labial feature, 0 to 19%, 20 to 39%, 40 to 59%, 60 to 79%, and 80 to 100%. These groupings, according to the single feature, labial place of articulation, were predicted by the overall distinctive feature profiles. The grouping of the 98 Modified Rhyme Test matrices according to the feature labiality showed remarkable confirmation of the feature-gram profiles. Table 9-2 shows that only four of the 98 cases deviated from predicted values. The cases on the diagonal of this discriminant analysis output confirm the strength of the initial grouping according to a given criterion. In Table 9-2, the 94 cases on the diagonal indicate agreement between the experimenters' grouping of cases according to the feature labiality and the grouping by the overall distinctive feature profiles. The relative degrees of importance of the predictor variables (features) can be found by the sequence of their entry in the stepwise analysis. The features were entered in the following order: 1) front/back place, 2) continuancy, 3) sonorancy, 4) voicing, 5) sibilancy, and 6) nasality. The *F* ratios associated with each of these features were significant.

Table 9-2. Discriminant analysis of 98 sets of Modified Rhyme Test data grouped by proportion of correct score on the feature labiality

Groups (based on %)	Number of cases classified by the discriminant analysis				
0–19	10	0	0	0	0
20–39	0	17	0	0	0
40–59	0	1	36	3	0
60–79	0	0	0	21	0
80–100	0	0	0	0	10

The procedures described above involving the initial grouping of the scores by the feature labiality were replicated for the other six features. The results were extremely compatible. It was concluded, then, that the distinctive feature errors of the Modified Rhyme Test can be grouped into five significantly different diagnostic categories. The feature-gram profiles of the five groups who were significantly different from each other are shown in Figures 9-5 to 9-9. These figures show the distinctive feature profiles of those groups of subjects whose labiality scores fell from 0 to 19%, 20 to 39%, 40 to 59%, 60 to 79%, and 80 to 100%, respectively. The subjects of each of these five groups exhibit significantly different error patterns.

The question, Why a feature-gram instead of traditional speech discrimination and/or articulation tests?, may be answered in part by viewing some inadequacies of traditional tests. It has been shown by Fry (1966), Danhauer and Singh (1975c), and Singh, Lawson, and Singh (1974) that in some cases the processing of phonemes by severely hard of hearing and deaf children cannot be predicted by pure tone audiograms. Although pure tone audiometry only tests the ear's sensitivity to specific single frequencies, speech processing is a special event dealing with complex signals that may have little correlation with processing of pure tones. Although audiometric techniques have attempted to overcome this inadequacy, they deal with percentage of discrimination scores, which do not provide sufficient insight into the interaction of the ear and the critical properties of the speech sounds. The percentage of correct speech discrimination score is unidimensional and, therefore, inadequate for the assessment of the multidimensional nature of the ear's response. Similar inadequacies are found in traditional speech articulation tests; they are also unidimensional and do not account for the multidimensional nature of speech production and errors in articulation.

DANHAUER AND SINGH (1975c): FEATURE-GRAM STUDY

The purpose in Danhauer and Singh (1975c) was to examine the speaking and listening performances of severely hearing-impaired individuals belonging to three different language groups. The speaking and listening performances were analyzed by the seven binary distinctive features: front/back place, labial place, sonorancy, nasality, continuancy, sibilancy, and voicing. The language groups selected were English, French, and Yugoslavian. The subjects whose speaking/listening behaviors were analyzed were young individuals with an average age of 8.77 years. The hearing sensitivity of the English-speaking subjects was never lower than 68 dB, for the Yugoslavian subjects never lower than 58 dB, and for the French subjects never lower than 69 dB.

Figure 9-10 shows, in histogram form, consonantal feature-grams for the American, Yugoslavian, and French subjects. It shows that the rank ordering of features and the percentage of values obtained for the features were similar for all three language groups. All three groups have the greatest amount of information transmitted by the features sonorancy, nasality, and voicing, and the least amount by the features place and labiality. These results show a striking similarity among the language groups for the magnitude of information transmission and ranking of features. Such a similarity was also noted by Singh and Black (1966), who used information transmission with 26 consonants as spoken and recognized by Hindi, Arabic, English, and Japanese subjects.

Figure 9-10 also shows that the feature-grams of the three hearing-impaired groups differ greatly from normal subjects. While all features have information transmission values of approximately 100% for the normal subject, the highest ranking feature scores (sonorancy and voicing) for any of the hearing-impaired groups did not exceed 33%. The lowest ranking feature, place, approached only 14%. The influence of the individual language backgrounds in this study has been minimized because of the utilization of "language-independent" feature criteria.

The fact that all three groups scored highest for sonorancy, nasality, and voicing may be explained by the audiograms. The residual hearing of the severely hearing-impaired subjects lies in the lower frequencies, and these features are processed in the low frequency domain. The audiograms do not account for the feature sibilancy, however. All three groups have poor hearing at all frequencies, especially above 2,000 Hz, where the information for the feature sibilancy lies. However, contrary to the audiometric prediction, sibilancy was an important feature for these subjects (see Chapter 5, discussion under *Klatt, 1968*).

SOME OTHER EXPERIMENTS: CASTING DOUBT ON DISTINCTIVE FEATURE THEORY

A number of experiments has been reported in the literature that casts doubt on the application of distinctive feature theory in processing speech sounds in certain domains. Two experiments, one reported by

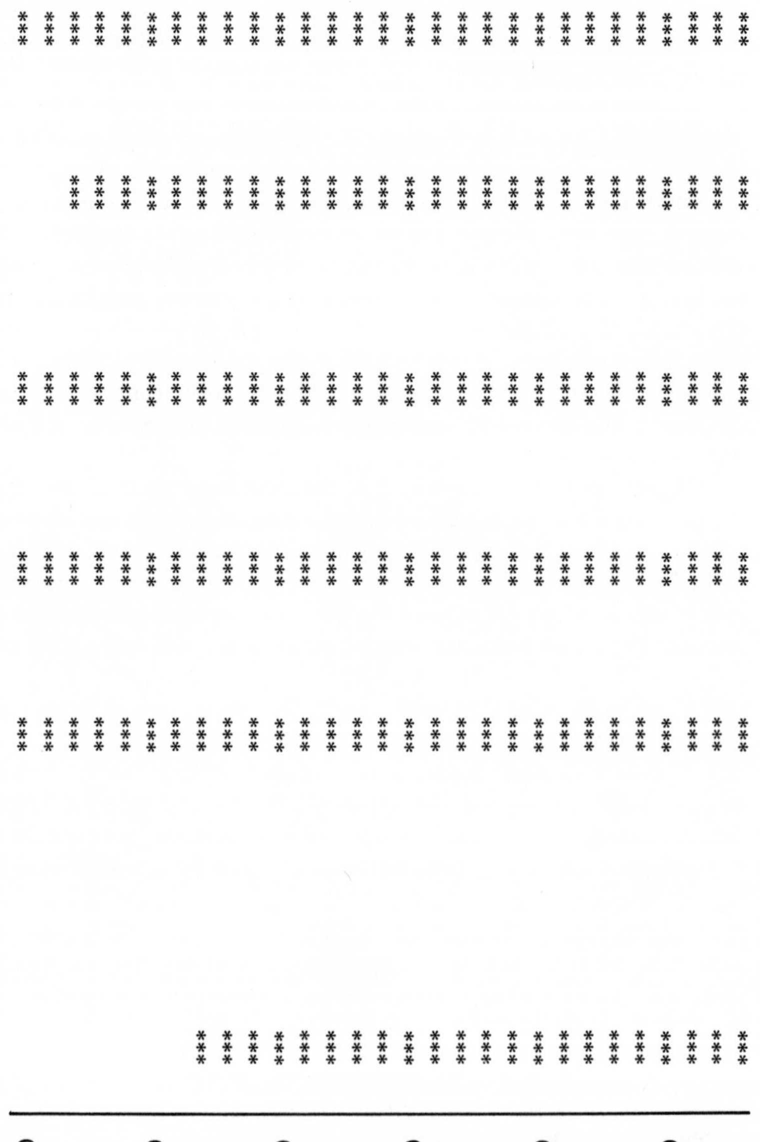
100
90
80
70
60
50
CORRECT PERCENTAGE

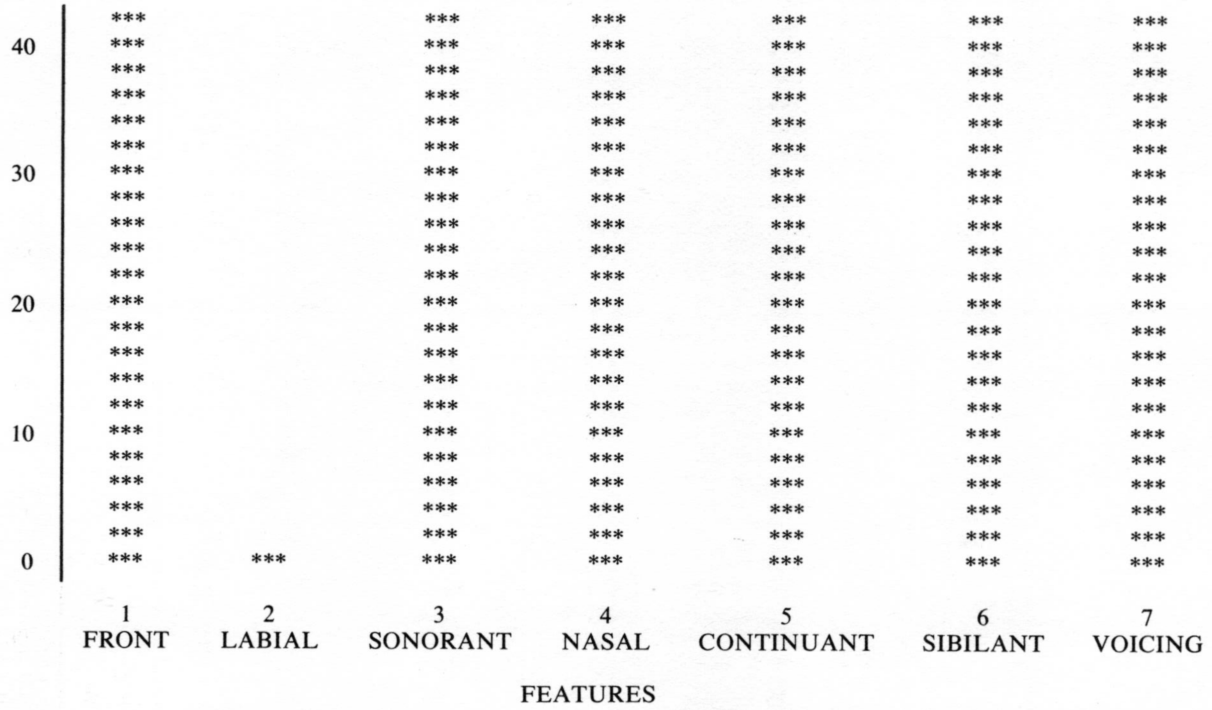

40

30

20

10

0

1 FRONT | 2 LABIAL | 3 SONORANT | 4 NASAL | 5 CONTINUANT | 6 SIBILANT | 7 VOICING

FEATURES

Figure 9-5. Feature profile for the 98 individual responses grouped according to 0 to 19% scores on the criterion of labial place.

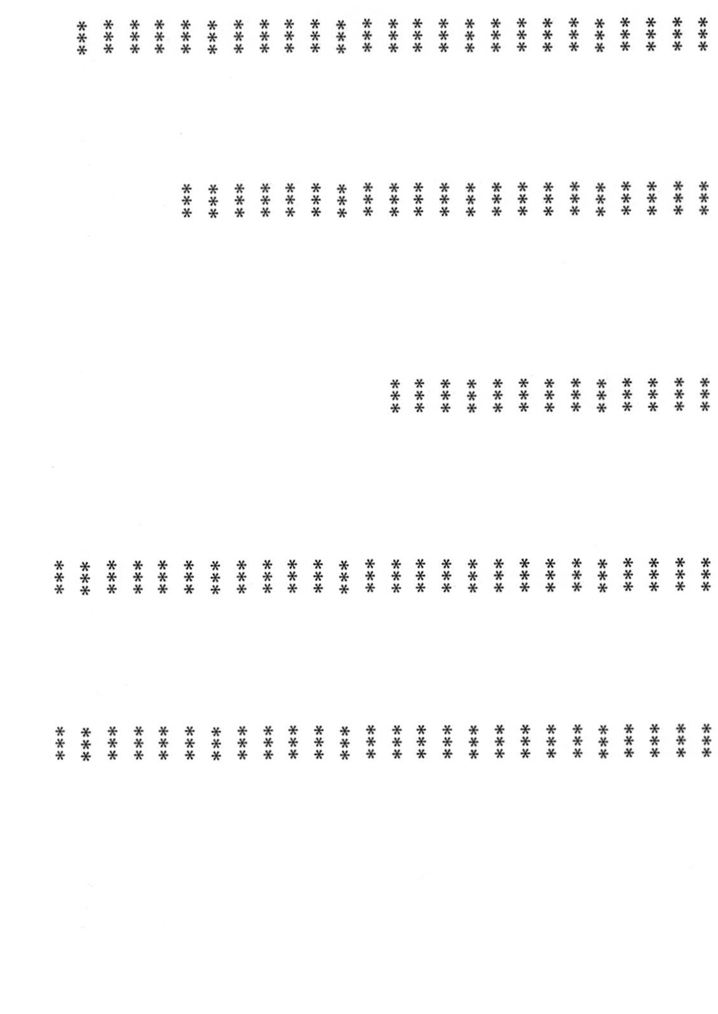

100 90 80 70 60 50

CORRECT PERCENTAGE

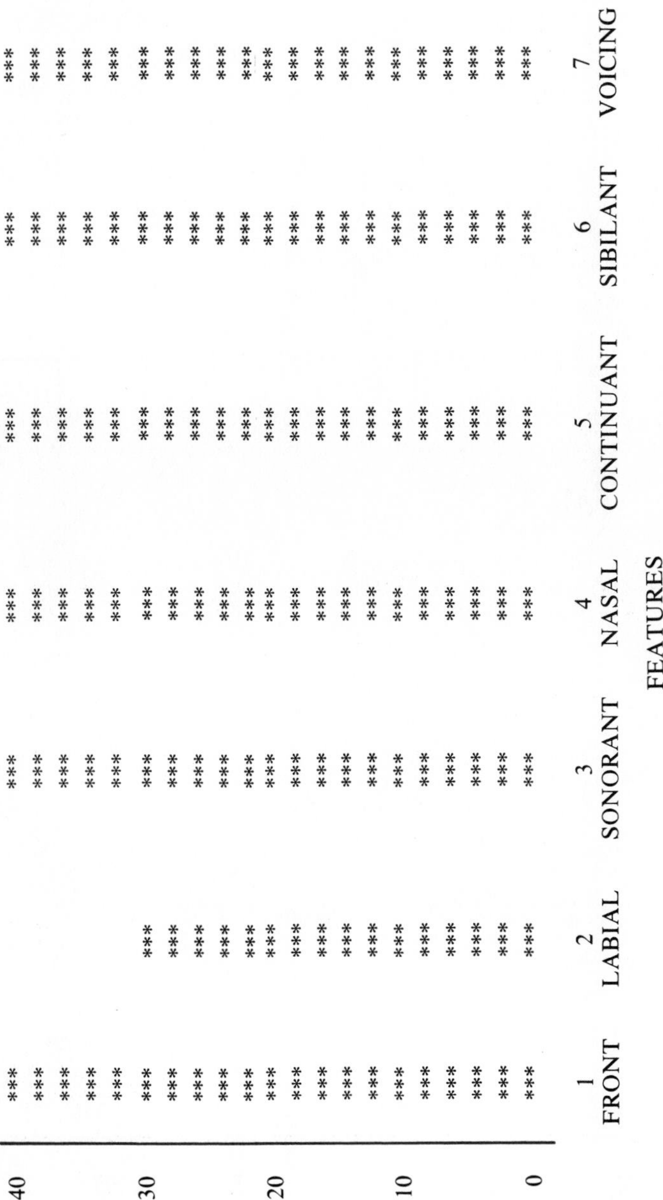

Figure 9-6. Feature profile for the 98 individual responses grouped according to 10 to 39% scores on the criterion of labial place.

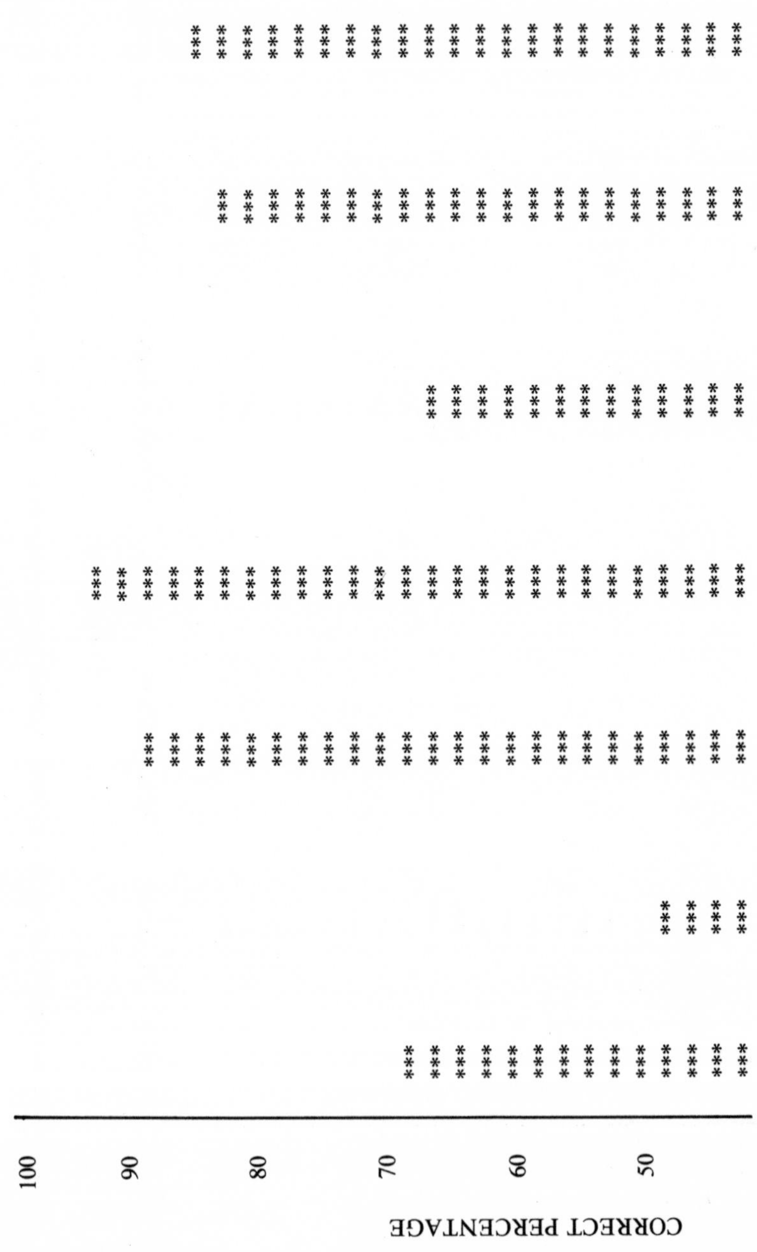
100
90
80
70
60
50
CORRECT PERCENTAGE

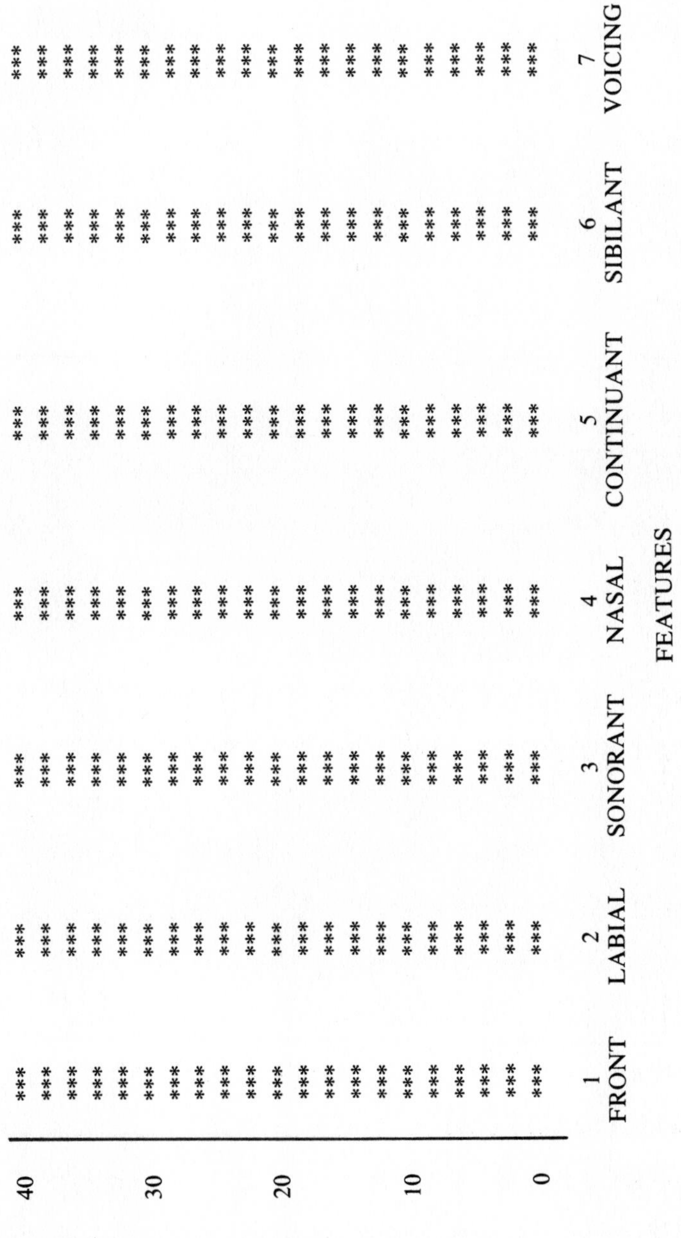

```
40 | ***    ***    ***    ***    ***    ***    ***
   | ***    ***    ***    ***    ***    ***    ***
   | ***    ***    ***    ***    ***    ***    ***
   | ***    ***    ***    ***    ***    ***    ***
   | ***    ***    ***    ***    ***    ***    ***
30 | ***    ***    ***    ***    ***    ***    ***
   | ***    ***    ***    ***    ***    ***    ***
   | ***    ***    ***    ***    ***    ***    ***
   | ***    ***    ***    ***    ***    ***    ***
   | ***    ***    ***    ***    ***    ***    ***
20 | ***    ***    ***    ***    ***    ***    ***
   | ***    ***    ***    ***    ***    ***    ***
   | ***    ***    ***    ***    ***    ***    ***
   | ***    ***    ***    ***    ***    ***    ***
   | ***    ***    ***    ***    ***    ***    ***
10 | ***    ***    ***    ***    ***    ***    ***
   | ***    ***    ***    ***    ***    ***    ***
   | ***    ***    ***    ***    ***    ***    ***
   | ***    ***    ***    ***    ***    ***    ***
   | ***    ***    ***    ***    ***    ***    ***
 0 | ***    ***    ***    ***    ***    ***    ***

      1      2        3        4         5          6         7
    FRONT  LABIAL  SONORANT  NASAL  CONTINUANT  SIBILANT  VOICING

                          FEATURES
```

Figure 9-7. Feature profile for the 98 individual responses grouped according to 40 to 59% scores on the criterion of labial place.

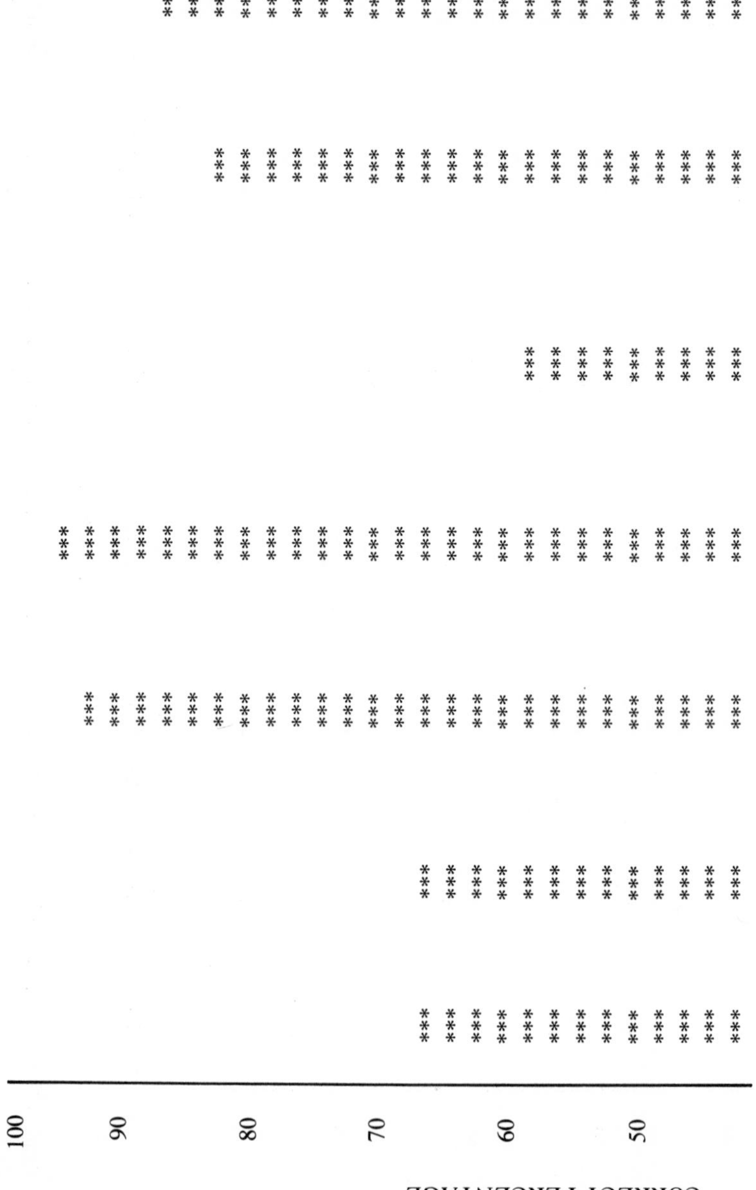
100
90
80
70
60
50
CORRECT PERCENTAGE

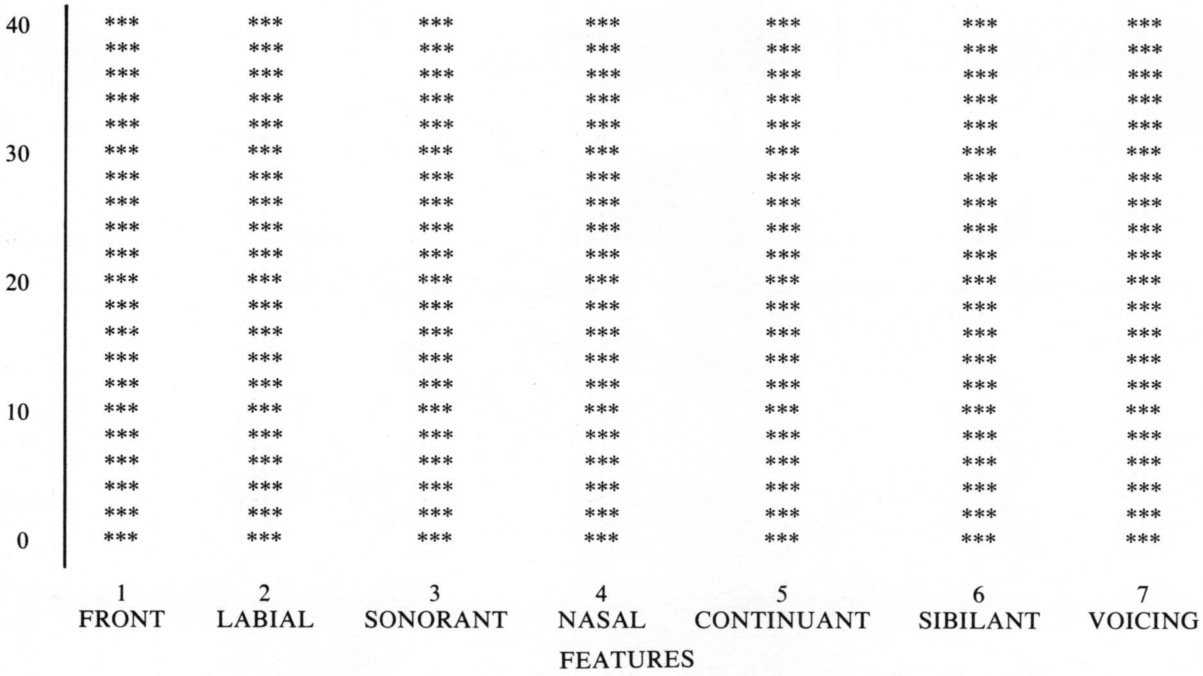

```
40 | ***   ***   ***   ***   ***   ***   ***
   | ***   ***   ***   ***   ***   ***   ***
   | ***   ***   ***   ***   ***   ***   ***
   | ***   ***   ***   ***   ***   ***   ***
   | ***   ***   ***   ***   ***   ***   ***
30 | ***   ***   ***   ***   ***   ***   ***
   | ***   ***   ***   ***   ***   ***   ***
   | ***   ***   ***   ***   ***   ***   ***
   | ***   ***   ***   ***   ***   ***   ***
   | ***   ***   ***   ***   ***   ***   ***
20 | ***   ***   ***   ***   ***   ***   ***
   | ***   ***   ***   ***   ***   ***   ***
   | ***   ***   ***   ***   ***   ***   ***
   | ***   ***   ***   ***   ***   ***   ***
   | ***   ***   ***   ***   ***   ***   ***
10 | ***   ***   ***   ***   ***   ***   ***
   | ***   ***   ***   ***   ***   ***   ***
   | ***   ***   ***   ***   ***   ***   ***
   | ***   ***   ***   ***   ***   ***   ***
   | ***   ***   ***   ***   ***   ***   ***
 0 | ***   ***   ***   ***   ***   ***   ***

      1      2        3        4         5          6         7
    FRONT  LABIAL  SONORANT  NASAL  CONTINUANT  SIBILANT  VOICING
                             FEATURES
```

Figure 9-8. Feature profile for the 98 individual responses grouped according to 60 to 79% scores on the criterion of labial place.

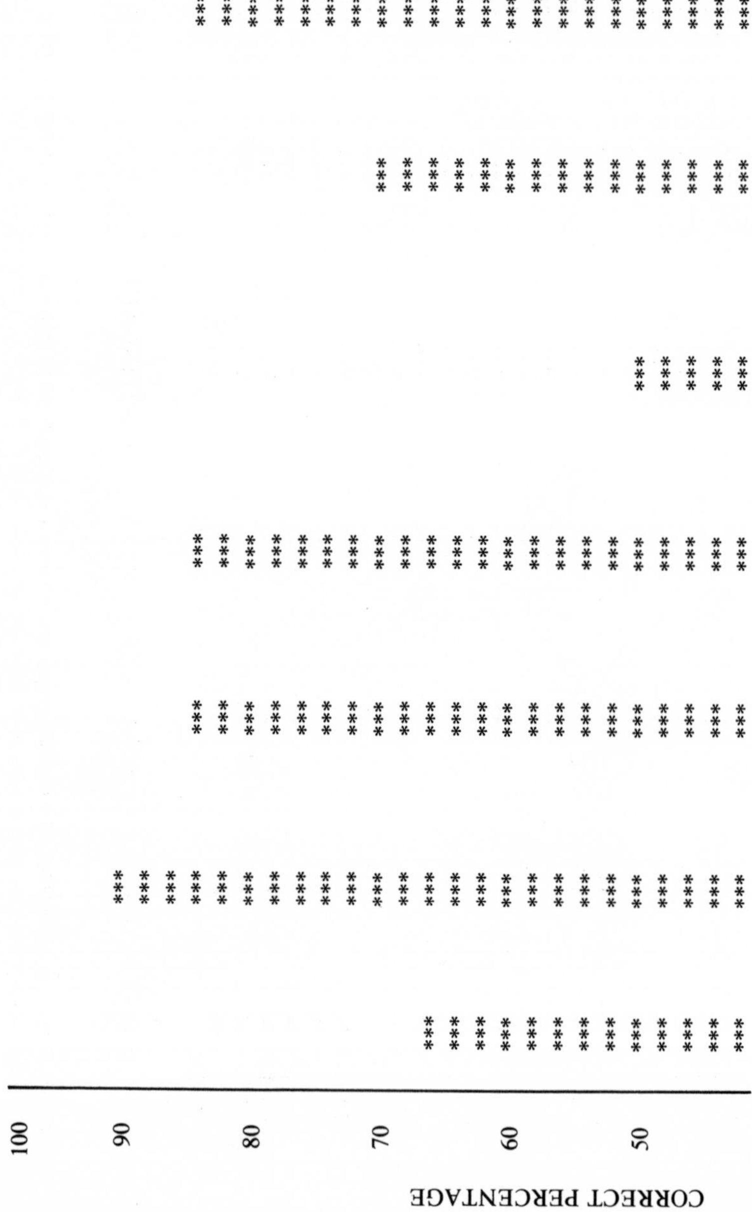
100
90
80
70
60
50
CORRECT PERCENTAGE

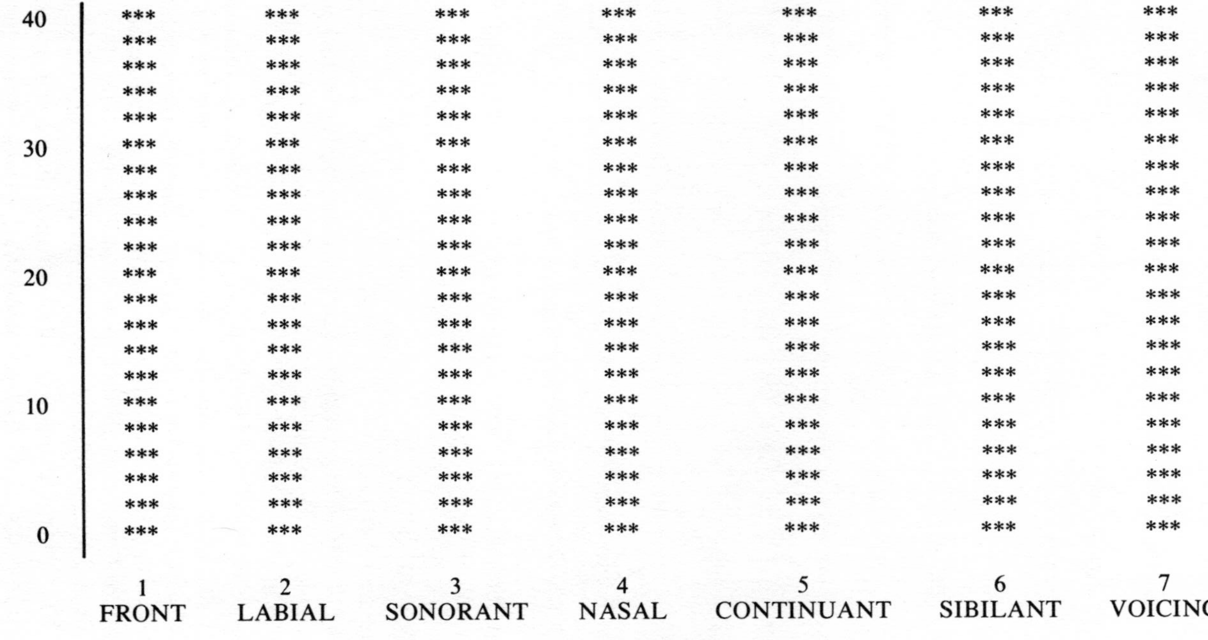

Figure 9-9. Feature profile for the 98 individual responses grouped according to 80 to 100% scores on the criterion of labial place.

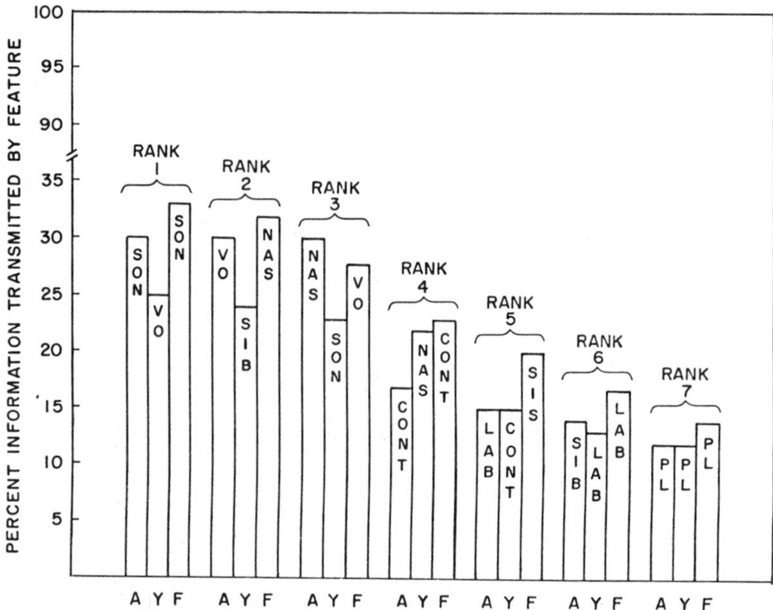

Figure 9-10. Feature-gram profiles, in histogram form, showing rank ordering and percentage of information transmitted by features for the American (A), Yugoslavian (Y), and French (F) subjects. (From Danhauer and Singh, 1975c.)

LaRiviere et al. (1974) and another reported by Ritterman and Freeman (1974), are included here.

LaRiviere et al. (1974)

LaRiviere and his colleagues (1974) conducted an experiment to investigate the conceptual reality of selected distinctive features. The features tested were: vocalicness, voicing, nasality, continuancy, and stridency. One hundred college students served as subjects, 20 for each of the features. Ten of the 20 subjects assigned to a given feature served in the control group and the other 10 served in the experimental group. The subjects were instructed to sort utterances into one of two categories. The difference between the experimental and the control groups was that the experimental group could solve this problem either in terms of paired associate memory or feature distinction, but the control group was allowed only the paired associate memory. LaRiviere et al. hypothesized that, if the criterion feature has conceptual reality, then the experimental group, who had feature categorization available in their task, would perform significantly better than the control group. For example, if the vocalic feature had conceptual reality, then the subjects would group /i, u, ɑ/ on the one side and /v, z, ʒ/ on another side. However, if the experimental group classified the phonemes in another way, it may be concluded that they did not utilize the concept of feature.

The result of this experiment is ambiguous, however, in the sense that three of the five features tested were found to have conceptual reality and the other two features were not found to have conceptual reality. The three features showing significant differences between the experimental and control conditions were stridency, vocalicness, and nasality. The two features exhibiting no significant differences between the experimental and control conditions were continuancy and voicing.

The reason for the lack of significant categorization for the continuancy and voicing features is probably attributable to the presence of a certain amount of confusion in the formulation of the test materials. The +continuant vs. the −continuant contrast failed to yield significantly different results because the −continuant consonant /tʃ/ was included in the +continuant category (see Table 2 of LaRiviere et al.). The mean percentage of correct score for the +continuant group, which included the consonants /tʃ, h, ʃ, v/, was 68.3, and for the −continuant group, which included the consonants /p, b, d, k/, was 60.1. It is intriguing that these authors included /tʃ/ in the +continuant group. Had they accepted the prevalent definition of /tʃ/ as being a −continuant consonant (Chomsky and Halle, 1968), the results might have been different. The result regarding lack of significant difference between the voiced and voiceless consonants cannot be explained.

Ritterman and Freeman (1974)

A group of college students was asked to respond to a list of consonant-vowel syllables. There were four groups of consonant-vowel syllables, one of which included tense consonants, another included lax consonants, the third included stop consonants, and the fourth group of syllables included continuant consonants. The results were analyzed in relation to the tallies of the number of trials necessary to learn the tense, lax, stop, and continuant features, on the one hand, and the number of errors committed on each of these features, on the other hand. The final outcome was that no significant difference was found either in the number of trials necessary to learn each of these feature specifications or in the number of errors made while learning these features.

The conclusion of this experiment is different from that of earlier experiments in that the features (e.g., voicing and continuancy) have shown differential weightings (Singh, 1971). The weighting of a given feature solely depends on the nature of the task (Singh, 1974). It is very probable that the task employed by Ritterman and Freeman was of such a nature that the differential weighting strategies generally associated with these two features were not evoked.

In discussing their results, Ritterman and Freeman use the LaRiviere et al. (1974) and Graham and House (1971) results, both of which cast doubt on the perceptual reality of distinctive features. It may be noted, however, that the Graham and House (1971) data were reanalyzed by Singh, Woods, and Tishman (1972), who had questioned the analysis technique used by Graham and House. (For discussion of this controversy, see Chapter 5 in this text). The reanalysis revealed the utilization of some important perceptual feature dimensions by the 4.5-year-old child.

References

Ahmed, R., and S. Agrawal. 1969. Significant features in the perception of (Hindi) consonants. J. Acoust. Soc. Amer. 45: 758–763.

Anglin, M. 1971. Perceptual space of English vowels in word context. Unpublished master's thesis, Howard University, Washington, D.C.

Berko, J., and R. Brown. 1960. Psycholinguistic research methods. *In* P. H. Mussen (ed.), Handbook of Research Methods. John Wiley & Sons, New York.

Black, J. W. 1957. Multiple-choice intelligibility tests. J. Speech Hear. Disord. 22: 213–235.

Black, J. W. 1970. Interconsonantal differences. *In* A. J. Bronstein, C. L. Shaver, and C. Stevens (eds.), Essays in Honor of Claude M. Wise, pp. 74–96. Standard Printing Co., Hannibal, Mo.

Blumstein, S., and W. Cooper. 1972. Identification versus discrimination of features in speech perception. Q. J. Exp. Psychol. 24: 207–214.

Blumstein, S., V. Tartter, and D. Michael. 1973. The role of distinctive features in the perception of vowels. In preparation.

Bricker, W. A. 1967. Errors in echoic behavior of pre-school children. J. Speech Hear. Res. 7: 67–76.

Brock, O. 1911. Slavische Phonetik. Carl Winter, Heidelberg.

Cairns, C. E. 1969. Markedness, neutralization, and universal redundancy rules. Language 45: 863–885.

Cairns, H., and C. Cairns. 1971. Linguistic Perspectives. *In* F. Williams (ed.), Analysis of Production Errors in the Phonetic Performance of School-Age Standard Speaking Children. Center for Communication Research, Austin, Texas.

Cairns, H. S., and F. Williams. 1972. An analysis of the substitution errors of a group of standard English-speaking children. J. Speech Hear. Res. 15: 811–820.

Carroll, J. D., and J. J. Chang. 1970. Analysis of individual differences in a multidimensional scaling via an n-way generalization of 'Eckart-Young' decomposition. Psychometrika 35: 283–319.

Chananie, J. D., and R. S. Tikofsky. 1969. Choice response time and distinctive features in speech discrimination. J. Exp. Psychol. 81: 161–163.

Chomsky, N., and M. Halle. 1968. The Sound Pattern of English, pp. 176–177 and 303–305. Harper & Row, New York.

Cole, R. A., and B. Scott. 1972. Distinctive feature control of decision time: Same-different judgments of simultaneously heard phonemes. Percept. Psychophys. 12: 91–94.

Compton, A. J. 1970. Generative studies of children's phonological disorders. J. Speech Hear. Disord. 35: 315–339.

Compton, A. J. 1975. Generative studies of children's phonological disorders: A strategy of therapy. *In* S. Singh (ed.), Measurement Procedures in Speech, Hearing, and Language, pp. 55–90. University Park Press, Baltimore.

Costello, J. Articulation instruction based on distinctive feature theory. In press.

Crocker, J. R. 1969. A phonological model of children's articulation competence. J. Speech Hear. Disord. 34: 203–213.

Crystal, T. H., and A. S. House. Local signal levels and differential performance in dichotic listening. *In* Proceedings of Speech Communication Seminars, Stockholm. Vol. 3, Speech Perception and Automatic Recognition. Almquist and Wiksell International, Stockholm, and John Wiley & Sons, New York. In press.

Danhauer, J. L. 1974. A multidimensional analysis of hearing impaired subjects' responses to sixteen consonants. Unpublished doctoral dissertation, Ohio University, Athens, Ohio.

Danhauer, J. L., and M. A. Appel. INDSCAL analysis of perceptual judgments for twenty-four consonants via visual, tactile, and visual-tactile sensory inputs. In press.

Danhauer, J. L., and S. Singh. 1973. A cross language study of speech production of children in audio-visual modalities. Acta Symbolica 4: 29–45.

Danhauer, J. L., and S. Singh. 1975a. Multidimensional Speech Perception by the Hearing Impaired. University Park Press, Baltimore. 130p.

Danhauer, J. L., and S. Singh. 1975b. A multidimensional scaling analysis of phonemic responses from hard of hearing and deaf subjects of three languages. Lang. Speech. 18: 42–64.

Danhauer, J. L., and S. Singh. 1975c. A study of "feature-gram" profiles for three different hearing impaired language groups. Scand. Audiol. 4: 67–71.

Day, R. S., and J. M. Vigorito. 1972. A parallel between degree of encodedness and the ear advantage: Evidence from a temporal order judgment task. Status Report on Speech Research, SR-31/32, pp. 41–47. Haskins Laboratories, New Haven, Conn.

Dixon, W. J., and F. J. Massey. 1969. Introduction to Statistical Analysis. McGraw-Hill, New York. 638p.

Elbert, M., R. L. Shelton, Jr., and W. B. Arndt. 1967. Development of a task for evaluation of articulation change. J. Speech Hear. Res. 10: 281–288.

Ervin-Tripp, S. M. 1966. Language development. *In* L. W. Hoffman and M. L. Hoffman (eds.), Review of Child Development, pp. 55–105. Russell Sage Foundation, New York.

Fant, G., U. Stålhammer, and I. Karlsson. 1974. Swedish vowels in speech material of various complexity. Presented at the Speech Communication Seminar, August 1–3, Stockholm.

Fry, D. B. 1966. The development of the phonological system in the normal and deaf child. *In* F. Smith and G. A. Miller (eds.), The Genesis of Language, pp. 187–206. MIT Press, Cambridge, Mass.

Graham, L., and A. House. 1971. Phonological oppositions in children: A perceptual study. J. Acoust. Soc. Amer. 49: 559–566.

Grant, M. 1971. INDSCAL Analysis of Hindi and English vowels. Unpublished master's thesis, Howard University, Washington, D.C.

Gupta, J. P., S. Agrawal, and R. Ahmed. 1969. Perception of (Hindi) consonants in clipped speech. J. Acoust. Soc. Amer. 45: 770–773.

Haas, W. 1963. Phonological analysis of a case of dyslalia. J. Speech Hear. Disord. 28: 239–245.

Halle, M. 1964. On the basis of phonology. *In* J. A. Fodor and J. J. Katz (eds), The Structure of Language: Readings in the Philosophy of Language, pp. 324–333. Prentice-Hall, Englewood Cliffs, N.J.

Hanson, G. 1967. Dimensions in speech sound perception: An experimental study of vowel perception. Ericsson Tech. 23: 3–175.

House, A. S., C. E. Williams, M. H. L. Hecker, and K. D. Kryter. 1965. Articulation testing methods: Consonantal differentiation with a closed-response set. J. Acoust. Soc. Amer. 37: 158–166.

Irwin, O. C. 1947a. Infant speech: Consonantal sounds according to manner of articulation. J. Speech Hear. Disord. 12: 402–404.

Irwin, O. C. 1947b. Infant speech: Consonantal sounds according to place of articulation. J. Speech Hear. Disord. 12: 397–401.

Jakobson, R. 1968. Child Language and Phonological Universals. Mouton, The Hague. (First published in 1941).

Jakobson, R., G. Fant, and M. Halle. 1951. Preliminaries to Speech Analysis: The Distinctive Features and Their Correlates. MIT Press, Cambridge, Mass. 58p.

Jeter, I., and S. Singh. 1972. A comparison of phonemic and graphemic features of eight English consonants in auditory and visual modes. J. Speech Hear. Res. 15: 201–210.

Johnson, S. C. 1967. Hierarchical clustering schemes. Psychometrika 32: 241–254.

Kamara, C., A. Kamara, and S. Singh. 1974. "Featuregram" analysis of articulation performance in various hearing and speech pathologies. Preprints of the Speech Communication Seminar, Stockholm (Aug. 1–3, 1974). Speech and Hearing Defects and Aids.

Kelly, D. H. 1973. Oral vibrotactile sensation: An evaluation of children exhibiting defective articulation. Unpublished doctoral dissertation, Ohio University, Athens, Ohio.

Kelly, D., and S. Singh. Prediction of articulation errors by a distinctive feature system. In preparation.

Kile, J. 1966. Predicting consonantal responses to filtered syllables. Unpublished doctoral dissertation, Ohio State University, Columbus, Ohio.

Klatt, D. 1968. Structure of confusions in short-term memory between English consonants. J. Acoust. Soc. Amer. 44: 401–407.

Kruskal, J. B. 1964a. Multidimensional scaling by optimizing goodness of fit to a nonmetric hypothesis. Psychometrika 29: 1–27.

Kruskal, J. B. 1964b. Nonmetric multidimensional scaling: A numerical method. Psychometrika 29: 115–129.

LaRiviere, C., H. Winitz, J. Reeds, and E. Herriman. 1974. The conceptual reality of selected distinctive features. J. Speech Hear. Res. 17: 122–133.

Leopold, W. E. 1947. Speech Development of a Bilingual Child. Vol. 2. Northwestern University Press, Evanston, Ill.

McGregor, L. V. 1972. An investigation of the perceptual structure of sixteen prevocalic English consonants embedded in sentential material. Unpublished doctoral dissertation, Ohio University, Athens, Ohio.

McReynolds, L., and S. Bennett. 1972. Distinctive feature generalization in articulation training. J. Speech Hear. Disord. 37: 461–470.

McReynolds, L. V., and K. Huston. 1971. A distinctive feature analysis of children's misarticulations. J. Speech Hear. Disord. 36: 155–166.

McReynolds, L. V., J. Kohn, and G. C. Williams. Articulatory defective children's discrimination of their production errors. J. Speech Hear. Disord. In press.

Menyuk, P. 1968. The role of distinctive features in children's acquisition of phonology. J. Speech Hear. Disord. 11: 138–146.

Menyuk, P. 1972. The Development of Speech. Bobbs-Merrill, New York.

Menyuk, P., and S. Anderson. 1969. Children's identification and reproduction of /w/, /r/, /l/. J. Speech Hear. Disord. 12: 39–52.

Messer, S. 1967. Implicit phonology in children. J. Verb. Learn. Verb. Behav. 6: 609–613.

Miller, G., and P. E. Nicely. 1955. An analysis of perceptual confusions among English consonants. J. Acoust. Soc. Amer. 27: 338–352.

Mitchell, L., and S. Singh. 1974. Perceptual structure of sixteen prevocalic English consonants sententially embedded. J. Acoust. Soc. Amer. 55: 1355–1357.

Nakazima, S. 1962. A comparative study of the speech developments of Japanese and American English in childhood. Stud. Phonol. 2: 17.

Oller, D. K. 1973. Regularities in abnormal child phonology. J. Speech Hear. Disord. 38: 36–47.

Peters, R. W. 1963. Dimensions of perception for consonants. J. Acoust. Soc. Amer. 35: 1985–1989.

Peterson, G. E., and H. I. Barney. 1952. Control methods used in the study of vowels. J. Acoust. Soc. Amer. 24: 175–184.

Pollack, E., and N. S. Rees. 1972. Disorders of articulation: Some clinical applications of distinctive feature theory. J. Speech Hear. Disord. 37: 451–461.

Pols, L. C. W., L. J. Van der Kamp, and R. Polmp. 1969. Perceptual and physical space of vowel sounds. J. Acoust. Soc. Amer. 46: 458–467.

Poole, I. 1934. Genetic development of articulation of consonant sounds in speech. Elem. English Rev. 11: 159–161.

Prather, E. M., D. L. Hedrick, and C. A. Kern. 1975. Articulation development in children aged 2 to 4 years. J. Speech Hear. Disord. 40: 179–191.

Pruzansky, S. 1970. Judgments of similarities among initial consonants using an auditory sorting apparatus. Presented at the 80th Meeting of the Acoustical Society of America, November 3–6, Houston.

Ritterman, S. I., and N. C. Freeman. 1974. Distinctive phonetic features as relevant and irrelevant stimulus dimensions in speech sound discrimination learning. J. Speech Hear. Res. 17: 417–425.

Shannon, C. E., and W. Weaver. 1963. The Mathematical Theory of Communication. University of Illinois Press, Urbana, Ill. 117p.

Shepard, R. N. 1962. The analysis of proximities: Multidimensional scaling with an unknown distance function. Psychometrika 27: 125–140, 219–246.

Shepard, R. N. 1972. Psychological representation of speech sounds. *In* E. E. David, Jr. and P. B. Denes (eds.), Human Communications: A Unified View, pp. 67–113. McGraw-Hill, New York.

Sievers, E. 1901. Grundzüge der Phonetik. Breitkopf und Härtel, Leipzig.

Singh, S. 1966. Cross-language study of perceptual confusion of plosive phonemes in two conditions of distortions. J. Acoust. Soc. Amer. 40: 635–656.

Singh, S. 1968. A distinctive feature analysis of responses to a multiple choice intelligibility test. Int. Rev. Appl. Linguist. 6: 37–53.

Singh, S. 1970a. Initially and transitionally truncated prevocalic English consonants spoken and recognized by native Hindi and English speakers. *In* A. Rosetti (ed.), Actes Du X Congrees International des Linguistes, pp. 245–255. Edition of the Socialist Republic of Rumania, Bucarest.

Singh, S. 1970b. Interrelationship of English consonants. *In* B. Hala, M. Romportl, and P. Janota (eds.), Proceedings of the Sixth International Congress of Phonetic Sciences, pp. 825–828. Publishing House of the Czechoslavak Academy of Sciences, Prague.

Singh, S. 1971. Perceptual similarities and minimal phonemic differences. J. Speech Hear. Res. 14: 113–124.

Singh, S. 1973. A unified theory of speech perception. Presented at the 1973 Annual Convention of American Speech and Hearing Association, October 10–15, Detroit.

Singh, S. 1974. A step toward a theory of speech perception. *In* Proceedings of Speech Communication Seminars, Stockholm. Vol. III, Speech Perception and Automatic Recognition. Almquist and Wiksell International, Stockholm, and John Wiley & Sons, New York.

Singh, S., and G. M. Becker. 1972. A comparison of four feature systems using data from three psychophysical methods. J. Speech Hear. Res. 15: 821–830.

Singh, S., and J. W. Black. 1966. Study of twenty-six intervocalic consonants as spoken and recognized by four language groups. J. Acoust. Soc. Amer. 39: 372–387.

Singh, S., J. W. Black, and E. Jancosek. Multidimensional analysis of the perceptual uniqueness of 31 English consonants. In press.

Singh, S., and R. Blackmon. 1974. Prediction of Rhyme test stimuli by a distinctive feature system. Unpublished Ohio University manuscript.

Singh, S., and D. C. Frank. 1972. A distinctive feature analysis of the consonantal substitution pattern. Lang. Speech 15: 109–218.

Singh, S., S. Faircloth, and M. A. Faircloth. Articulatory proficiency in the conversational speech of mentally retarded subjects. J. Speech Hear. Res. In press.

Singh, S., G. Lawson, and K. Singh. 1974. Feature prediction of the modified Rhyme test in grouping of hearing impaired subjects according to the uniqueness of their errors. Presented at the 1974 ASHA meeting, Las Vegas.

Singh, S., and S. B. Polen. 1972. The use of a distinctive feature model in speech pathology. Acta Symbolica 3: 17–35.

Singh, S., and K. Singh. 1972a. A search for the perceptual features of 29 prevocalic Hindi consonants. Presented at the 83rd Meeting of the Acoustical Society of America, April 18–21, Buffalo.

Singh, S., and K. S. Singh. 1972b. A self generating distinctive feature model for diagnosis prognosis and therapy. Acta Symbolica 3: 88–99.

Singh, S., and D. R. Woods. 1971. Perceptual structure of 12 American English vowels. J. Acoust. Soc. Amer. 49: 1861–1866.

Singh, S., and D. R. Woods. 1972. Implication of the Perception of similarities for phonetic theory. *In* A. Rigualt and R. Charbonneau (eds.), Proceedings of the 7th International Congress of Phonetic Sciences, pp. 608–612. Mouton, The Hague.

Singh, S., D. R. Woods, and G. M. Becker. 1972. Perceptual structure of 22 prevocalic English consonants. J. Acoust. Soc. Amer. 52: 1698–1713.

Singh, S., D. R. Woods, and A. Tishman. 1972. An alternative MD-SCAL analysis of the Graham and House data. J. Acoust. Soc. Amer. 51: 666–668.

Snow, K. 1963. A detailed analysis of the articulation responses of normal first grade children. J. Speech Hear. Disord. 6: 277–290.

Stevens, K. N., and A. S. House. 1972. Speech Perception. *In* J. V. Tobias (ed.), Foundations of Modern Auditory Theory, pp. 1–62. Academic Press, New York.

Studdert-Kennedy, M., and D. Shankweiler. 1970. Hemispheric specialization for speech perception. J. Acoust. Soc. Amer. 48: 579–594.

Tannahill, J. C., and L. V. McReynolds. 1972. Consonant discrimination as a function of distinctive feature differences. J. Aud. Res. 12: 101–108.

Templin, M. 1957. Certain Language Skills in Children. University of Minnesota Institute of Child Welfare Monograph No. 26.

Templin, M. C., and F. L. Darley. 1969. The Templin-Darley Tests of Articulation. 2nd Ed. The University of Iowa, Iowa City, Iowa.

Terbeek, D., and R. Harshman. 1971. Crosslanguage differences in the perception of natural vowel sounds. UCLA Working Papers in Phonetics.

Torgerson, W. S. 1958. Theory and Method of Scaling. John Wiley & Sons, New York. 460p.

Van Riper, C., and J. V. Irwin. 1958. Voice and Articulation. Prentice-Hall, Englewood Cliffs, N.J.

Voelker, C. H. 1945. Technique for a phonetic frequency distribution count in formal English speech. Extrait Arch. Neelandaises Phonetique Experimentale 11: 69–72.

Walden, B. E., and A. A. Montgomery. 1973. Dimensions of consonant perception in normal and hearing impaired listeners. Presented at the 1973 Annual Convention of the American Speech and Hearing Association, October 10–15, Detroit.

Wang, M., and R. C. Bilger. 1973. Consonant confusions in noise: A study of perceptual features. J. Acoust. Soc. Amer. 54: 1248–1266.

Weber, J. L. 1970. Patterning of deviant articulation behavior. J. Speech Hear. Disord. 35: 135–141.

Weiner, F. F., and S. Singh. 1974. Multidimensional analysis of choice reaction time judgments on pairs of English fricatives. J. Exp. Psychol. 102: 615–620.

Weir, R. H. 1962. Language in the Crib. Mouton, The Hague.

Wellman, B. L., I. M. Case, I. G. Mengert, and D. E. Bradbury. 1931. Speech sounds of young children. Univ. Iowa Stud. Child Welfare 5 (no. 2).

Wickelgren, W. A. 1966. Distinctive features and errors in short-term memory for English consonants. J. Acoust. Soc. Amer. 39: 388–398.

Wilson, K. V. 1963. Multidimensional analysis of confusions of English consonants. Amer. J. Psychol. 76: 89–95.

Winer, B. 1971. Statistical Principles in Experimental Design. McGraw-Hill, New York. 907p.

Wise, C. 1958. Introduction to Phonetics. Prentice-Hall, Englewood Cliffs, N.J.

Wish, M. 1970. An INDSCAL analysis of the Miller and Nicely consonant confusion data. Presented at the 80th Meeting of the Acoustical Society of America, November 3–6, Houston.

Index

Ahmed and Agrawal, nonsense syllable test, 115–116
Alveolarity, 6
Anglin, analysis of vowel perception, 84, 86
Anterior feature
  in different feature systems, 97–98
  errors in, 183–184
Aperture, articulatory gesture, 99
Articulation
  development of, in children, 174–175
  places of
    alveolar, 6
    bilabial, 5–6
    and children's speech errors, 18
    in different feature systems, 90–95
    in Miller and Nicely system, 44
    as ternary feature system, 19
    and tongue, 19
    in Singh and Black consonant system, 51
    velar, 6
  study of errors, 170–171
Articulation development, explanation by rules and feature sets, 207–208
Articulation deviation
  clinical application of distinctive features to, 228–229
  definition of, 205
  distinctive feature analysis of, 213–214
  distinctive feature rules for describing, 218
  in dyslexic child, 206
  and feature generalization, 214–215
  feature-gram in diagnosis of, 218–222
  interpretation with distinctive feature system, 226
  measuring and treating, 231
  and phoneme substitution, 215–218
    manner substitution, 216, 217
    place substitution, 216, 217
    principles governing, 217
  phonemic, and distinctive feature error, 210–213
  role of distinctive features in, 209–210
  and speech discrimination, 230–231
  therapeutic strategy for, 208–209
  transfer of training, 206–207
  use of Templin-Darley test, 223–226
Articulation therapy, 16

Back feature
  in different feature systems, 98–99
  errors in, 189–191
Bilabiality, 5–6
Binary feature, definition of, 6
Bricker, study of phoneme acquisition, 166–167

Cairns and Williams, study of phoneme acquisition, 170–171
Chomsky and Halle, consonant feature system of
  anterior/nonanterior, 59–60

Chomsky and Halle, consonant feature system of—*continued*
  application of, 63–66
  cavity features in, 58–62
  consonantal/nonconsonantal, 58
  continuant/noncontinuant, 62–63
  coronal/noncoronal, 59
  distributed/nondistributed, 60–62
  glottal constrictions in, 62
  major class features of, 57–58
  manner of articulation features in, 62–63
  release features in, 63
  rounding in, 60
  secondary apertures in, 62
  sonorant/nonsonorant, 58
  strident/nonstrident, 63
  tense/nontense, 63
  tongue body features of
    back/nonback, 60
    high/nonhigh, 60
    low/nonlow, 60
  universal phonetic features of, 57
  vocalic/nonvocalic, 58
  voicing in, 63
Chomsky and Halle, vowel feature system of
  back/round, 82–83
  high/low, 82
  and Singh-Woods perceptual analysis, 85–86
Compact feature in different feature systems, 97–98
Competence
  description of, 29
  distinguished from performance, 29–31
Compton
  analysis of distinctive features and articulation problems, 209–210, 226–228
  clinical application of distinctive feature analysis, 228–229
  hypothesis of normal phonological development, 229
  phonological theory of, 230
Confusion matrix, 41, 69
Consonants
  perception of, 34
  production of, 33
Consonant features
  affrication, 42
  anterior/nonanterior, 59
  compact/diffuse, 37, 47
  consonantal/nonconsonantal, 37, 45, 58
  continuant/interrupted, 38, 47, 62
  coronal/noncoronal, 59
  duration, 42, 51
  frication, 49
  grave/acute, 38, 47
  liquid, 51
  nasal/oral, 38, 44, 47, 49, 62
  sonorant/nonsonorant, 58
  strident/mellow, 39, 63
  tense/lax, 38, 63
  vocalic/nonvocalic, 35, 45, 58
  voicing, 42, 47, 49, 63
Consonant feature systems. *see also under* specific researchers
  Chomsky and Halle, 55–66
  Halle, 44–48
  Jakobson, Fant, and Halle, 34–40
  Miller and Nicely, 41–44
  multidimensional analysis of, 69–72
  problems with, 66–69
  Singh and Black, 48–52
  "true" perceptual, 69–72
  Wickelgren, 52–55
Consonant perception
  dichotic listening tasks for, 124–127
  feature studies on, 101–123
    test for natural perceptual categories, 119–123
    using acoustic distortion, 102–105
    using acoustic and linguistic distortions, 107–112
    using cross-linguistic settings, 105–107
    using nonsense syllables, 115–118
    using short-term memory recall, 113–114
    using similarity judgments, 114–115

using stimulus-response choice, 118–119
using truncated consonants, 112–113
theory of, 145
Contact (occlusion) in Halle consonant system, 45
Continuancy
in different feature systems, 95–96, 99
errors in, 198–200
Coronal feature
in different feature systems, 97–98
errors in, 184–187
Costello, measurement and treatment of misarticulation, 231
Crocker, theory of feature sets, 207–208

Delayed release errors, 196–198
Dichotic listening tasks, role of distinctive features in, 124–127
Disparities
distinctive feature, 10
phonemic, 10
Distinctive feature count vs. phoneme count, 16–17
Distinctive feature disparities, 10
Distinctive feature matrix, 6–9
Distinctive feature model, application of to speech therapy, 22
Distinctive feature theory, doubts about, 241, 252–254
Distinctive features
a posteriori retrieval of, 127–144
clinical application of, 228–229
as criterion for phonemic development, 178–204
definition of, 5
role in dichotic listening tasks, 124–127
use of, in children's misarticulations, 226–228
used to predict speech discrimination tests, 233–241
Distinctive feature systems
a posteriori, 127
a priori, 102
in prediction of perceptual responses, 123
use of INDSCAL with, 131–144
Distributed error, 191–193
Duration in different feature systems, 97

Elbert, Shelton, and Arndt, training for articulation production, 206–207

Feature, concept of, 4
Feature acquisition, method for evaluating, 178–204
Feature errors, study of in normally developing children, 178–204
anterior, 183–184
back, 189–191
comparison in pre- and postvocalic positions, 202–203
continuant, 198–200
coronal, 184–187
delayed release, 196–198
distributed, 191–193
features having highest error, 203
high, 187–189
lateral, 195–196
nasal, 193–195
voice, 200–202
Feature-gram
description, 219
study, 240–241
Feature set, defined, 208
Fricatives
proportion of errors in production of, 183–204
Fundamental source feature of Jakobson, Fant, and Halle, 37

Glide feature in different feature systems, 99
Grave feature in different feature systems 97–98
Gupta, Agrawal, and Ahmed, nonsense syllable test, 116–118

Haas, study of articulation in dyslexic child, 206
Halle
  consonant feature system of
    application of, 48
    consonantal, 45
    continuant, 47
    diffuse, 47
    grave, 47
    nasal, 47
    strident, 47
    vocalic, 45
    voiced, 47–48
  see also Chomsky and Halle, and Jakobson, Fant, and Halle
High feature
  in different feature systems, 98–99
  errors in, 187–189

INDSCAL feature system (Singh, Woods, and Becker), 72–74
INDSCAL retrieval of distinctive features, 131–144
Inequality
  interfeature, 22, 24–28
  intrafeature, 22–24
Interfeature inequality, 22, 24–28
Intrafeature inequality, 22–24
Irwin, O. C., study of phonene acquisition in infancy, 161–164
Irwin, R., study of speech perception and production in children, 172–174

Jakobson's hypothesis of phonological acquisition, 156–157
Jakobson, Fant, and Halle
  consonant feature system, 34–40
    compact/diffuse, 37
    consonantal/nonconsonantal, 37
    continued/interrupted, 38–39
    fundamental source feature, 37
    grave/acute, 38
    hierarchy of, 39–40
    nasal/oral, 38
    resonance feature, 37
    secondary consonantal source feature, 38–39
    strident/mellow, 39
    supplemental resonator feature, 38
    tense/lax, 38
    tonality feature, 38
    vocalic/nonvocalic, 35–37
  vowel feature system of
    compact/diffuse, 78
    grave/acute, 78

Kamara, Kamara, and Singh, use of feature-gram, 218–222
Kelly, use of Templin-Darley test, 223–226

Language acquisition. *see* Phonological acquisition
Lateral errors, 195–196
Liquid feature, in different feature systems, 99

McDonald Deep Test, 212–213, 230
McReynolds and Bennett, study of feature generalization and misarticulation, 214–215
McReynolds and Huston, study of misarticulation and feature error, 210–213
McReynolds, Kohn, and Williams, study of speech discrimination, 230–231
Markedness
  definition of, 25–26
  and feature error, 203–204
  role in phoneme acquisition, 160, 175–178
Matrix
  confusion, 41, 69
  distinctive feature, 6–9
Menyuk, study of phoneme acquisition, 167–169
Menyuk and Anderson, study of identification and reproduction of speech sounds, 169–170

Messer, study of phoneme acquisition, 167
Miller and Nicely
  confusion matrix of, 41
  consonant feature system of
    affrication in, 42–44
    compared with Jakobson, Fant, and Halle, 41–42
    duration in, 42
    nasality in, 44
    place of articulation in, 44
    voicing in, 42
  feature study of perception, 102–105
Multiple Choice Intelligibility Test, 51–52

Nakazima, study of phoneme acquisition, 164
Nasality
  compared to voicing, 90
  errors in, 193–195
Natural class, definition of, 11

Occlusion (contact) in Halle consonant system, 45
Oller, demonstration of distinctive feature rules describing misarticulation, 218
Openness feature in different feature systems, 99

Perceptual features, independence of, 144–145
Perceptual feature system, 83–87
Perceptual responses predicted by feature systems, 123
Performance and competence, 29–31
Peterson and Barney, vowel feature system of, 78–80
Phoneme count vs. distinctive feature count, 16–17
Phoneme distinctions, classification of, 9–11
Phonemes
  articulatory and acoustic properties of, 3
  definition of, 3
  determining feature specification of, 5–6
  differences between, 5
  dissimilarity hierarchy, 11–15
  interrelationships of, 11
  magnitude of differences between, 21
  maximally similar pair of, 8
  minimally distinct pair of, 8
  number of, in English, 32
  perception of, 101
Phonemic system, definition of concept of, 4–5
Phonemically minimal pair, 10
Phonetic features
  acquisition in children, 178–204
  anterior, 183–184
  articulatory description of, 180
  coronal, 184–187
  having highest proportion of error, 203
  high, 187–189
Phonetic feature system of Weiner and Bernthal, 179
Phonological acquisition
  age of, 157–159
  age of 100% correct production, 159–160
  analysis of substitution errors during, 167
  in children
    vs. adults
    study of articulation errors in, 170–171, 174–175
    study of domain of speech production and perception, 172–174
  indentification and reproduction of speech sounds in, 169–170
  in infancy, 164
  Jakobson's hypothesis of, 156–157
  role of distinctive features in, 167–169
  study of,
    in infancy, 161–164

Phonological acquisition –*continued*
in preschoolers, 166–167
in spontaneous speech of retarded, 171–172
using picture vocabulary articulation test, 165
Phonological development
of child, 23–24
normal
hypothesis of, 229
related to deviant development, 229–230
Phonological disorders, Compton's theory of acquisition of, 230
Phonological feature system of Chomsky and Halle, 80–83
Pollack and Rees, analysis of distinctive features and articulation, 213–214
Poole, study of phoneme acquisition, 159–160, 161
Prather, Hedrick, and Kern, study of articulation development in children, 174–175
Pre- and postvocalic positions, influence on feature errors, 202–203

Resonance feature of Jakobson, Fant, and Halle, 37
Retroflex feature in different feature systems, 99

Secondary consonantal source feature, 38–39
Shepard, analysis of confusion matrices by, 83–84
Similarity count, 29–30
Similarity matrix, defined, 69
Singh
similarity judgment study of consonant perception, 114–115
stimulus-response test of consonant perception, 118–119
study of distortion and consonant perception, 107–112
study of truncated consonants and perception, 112–113
Singh and Black
consonant feature system of
duration in, 51
extension of, 51–52
frication in, 49
liquid consonants in, 51
and Miller and Nicely system, 48–49
nasality in, 49
place of articulation in, 51
voicing in, 49
feature study of perception, 105–107
Singh, Faircloth, and Faircloth, study of spontaneous speech of retarded, 171–172
Singh and Frank, study of phoneme substitution, 215–218
Singh and Woods, analysis of vowel perception, 84–87
Singh, Woods, and Becker, INDSCAL feature system of, 71–74
Snow, study of phoneme acquisition, 165
Sonorants, proportion of errors in production of, 183–204
Speaker problems
counting errors in, 16–17
sample, 13–15
Speech
perception of, 3
production of, 3
Speech discrimination tests
inadequacies of tranditional, 240–241
Modified Rhyme Test, 235–240
multiple choice intelligibility, 233–234
same/different discrimination tasks, 234
Speech perception, assessment of, 233–241
Stops
in different feature systems, 99
proportion of errors in production of, 183–204

Stridency, in different feature systems, 96
Supplemental resonator feature, 38

Templin, study of phoneme acquisition, 160–161
Templin-Darley Diagnostic Test of Articulation, 223
Ternary feature, 6
Therapy, sample strategies for, 28
Tonality feature of Jakobson, Fant, and Halle, 38
Tongue and places of articulation, 19
Tree diagram, use of, 12–13

Unnatural class, definition of, 11

Velarity, 6
Voicing
  compared to nasality, 90
  in different feature systems, 96–97
  errors in, 25, 200–202
Vowel features
  back/rounded, 82
  compact/diffuse, 78
  grave/acute, 78
  high/low, 82
  tense/lax, 77
Vowel feature systems
  Jakobson, Fant, and Halle, 77–78
  perceptual, 83–87
  Peterson and Barney, 78–80
  phonological, of Chomsky and Halle, 80–83
Vowel perception
  a posteriori features of, 147–152
  confusion matrix of, 151
  cross-linguistic, 150–151
  Hindi-English, 151–152
  multidimensional scaling of, 147, 148–149
  of natural and synthesized vowels, 147
  theory of, 84–87
Vowels
  articulatory description of, 75–77
  perception of, 34
  production of, 33

Weber, therapeutic strategy for articulation problems, 208–209
Weiner and Bernthal, study of phonetic feature acquisition, 178–204
Wellman, study of phoneme acquisition, 157–159, 161
Wickelgren
  consonant feature system of
    and Halle system, 52–55
    and Jakobson Fant, and Halle system, 52
    and Miller and Nicely system, 52–55
    openness, defined in, 55
  feature study of perception, 113–114